# A DOCTOR'S DOZEN

Catherine Florio Pipas MD, MPH

# A DOCTOR'S DOZEN

. . . . . . . . . . .

## TWELVE STRATEGIES

## FOR PERSONAL HEALTH

## AND A CULTURE

## OF WELLNESS

Dartmouth College Press | Hanover, New Hampshire

613.2
Pip

Dartmouth College Press

An imprint of University Press of New England

www.upne.com

© 2018 Trustees of Dartmouth College

All rights reserved

Manufactured in the United States of America

Designed by Mindy Basinger Hill

Typeset in Calluna Pro

For permission to reproduce any of the material in this book, contact Permissions, University Press of New England, One Court Street, Suite 250, Lebanon NH 03766; or visit www.upne.com

Library of Congress Cataloging-in-Publication Data

*Names*: Pipas, Catherine Florio, author.

*Title*: A doctor's dozen: twelve strategies for personal health and a culture of wellness / Catherine Florio Pipas, MD, MPH.

*Description*: Hanover, New Hampshire: Dartmouth College Press, [2018] | Includes bibliographical references and index.

*Identifiers*: LCCN 2018007865 (print) | LCCN 2018012231 (ebook) | ISBN 9781512603002 (epub, pdf, & mobi) | ISBN 9781512602999 (paperback: alk. paper)

*Subjects*: LCSH: Health—Popular works. | Mind and body—Popular works. | Nutrition—Popular works. | Self-care, Health—Popular works.

*Classification*: LCC RA773 (ebook) | LCC RA773 .P57 2018 (print) | DDC 613.2—dc23

LC record available at https://lccn.loc.gov/2018007865

5  4  3  2  1

THIS BOOK IS DEDICATED TO MY TEACHERS:

MY PATIENTS, MY STUDENTS, AND MY FAMILY.

I have learned so much from all of you, and

I am grateful for this opportunity to give back.

If there is anything I have learned about men and women,
it is that there is a deeper [positive] spirit than is ever evident.
Just as the rivers we see are minor compared to the underground streams, so, too, the idealism that is visible is minor
compared to what people carry in their hearts unreleased or
scarcely released. Mankind is waiting and longing for those
who can accomplish the task of untying what is knotted, and
bringing these underground waters to the surface.

ALBERT SCHWEITZER

# CONTENTS

# PREFACE

In 2011 I attended Dartmouth's medical-school graduation, but that year I marched not with faculty but with the graduates, receiving an MPH degree. I sat among aspiring physicians and scientists, celebrating, reflecting, and eager to be congratulated and inspired by our speakers. The messages were broad, clear, and directed: achievement in academics, innovation in science, contribution to society, commitment to global populations, improvement of health-care systems, and alleviation of social injustice. The themes continued on and on: lead change, transform the world, be more than possible, do more than ever.

As expectations for "more" broadcast from microphones, I looked around into the eyes of students whom I knew well. I saw colleagues who were not sleeping, exercising, or eating healthily; who were missing their families and feeling unenergized, disillusioned, disengaged, and in some cases depressed and desperate to come off medication they had hoped to prescribe only for patients. Looking around, I felt an urge to stand up and shout, "What about us?" Don't we need to be told to care for ourselves, look after one another, prioritize our own well-being? Don't we, in our profession, want to emphasize that our impact on society depends not only on our ability to care for patients, conduct research, and teach but also on our ability to prioritize self-care, sustain personal well-being, and model wellness for others? At that moment I envisioned this book for my students and colleagues.

*A Doctor's Dozen* is a collection of lessons I have learned from patients and colleagues on my own journey toward wellness and my quest to promote health and self-care in others. The setting is my office, and I invite you to come and see what I have seen, hear what I have heard, feel what I have felt, and learn what I have learned. I introduce you to my patients, including health professionals, across all phases of life, with a range of health challenges and unique personal stories.

Achieving a healthy life comes from knowing ourselves, prioritizing personal wellness, and embracing change. The twelve lessons are organized into three parts: "Self-Awareness," "Self-Care," and "Self-Improvement," with four lessons in each part. Each lesson is illustrated by a patient's story, backed by science and linked to a strategy that anyone could apply. *A Doctor's Dozen* can be read and applied continuously or used as a monthly toolbox, focusing on one strategy at a time over the course of a year.

Personal wellness is a gift to oneself and to others. *A Doctor's Dozen* is my gift to you on your journey to the healthiest life possible. I hope that in reading this book you will learn as I have from others' successes and challenges, apply these twelve strategies to yourself, and advance your pursuit of health. I congratulate you for making a commitment to your own wellness and thank you for advancing my vision of healthy individuals contributing to healthy communities.

# A DOCTOR'S DOZEN

. . . . . . . . . . . .

# THE TWENTY-FIRST-CENTURY HEALTH CONUNDRUM

The quest for health transcends age, time, and culture and is vital to personal performance and societal success. Health affects life and is critical to each of us in our roles as parent, child, spouse, teacher, mentor, and citizen. The health and sustainability of a team, an organization, and a nation depend on and are determined by the health of each of their members. Strengthening the quality of health within a population requires prioritizing the health of every individual. Healthy individuals who model healthy behaviors create healthier communities.

For the first time in history, the current generation of young adults in our nation is less healthy than their parents. Individuals in today's society face new and different health threats from those of a century ago, and twenty-first-century health challenges are highly linked to personal health behavior.[1] Health outcomes across our nation are unacceptable and are complicated by a complex and culturally diverse environment. The United States is ranked seventeenth among developed countries in life expectancy, a global outcome and measure of a population's overall health, despite the fact that we spend more per capita on health care than any country in the world.

Achievements driven by those in the fields of research, public health, medicine, and medical technology have led to a thirty-year gain in life expectancy, from 47 to 77 years between 1900 and 2000. The development and distribution of vaccines, antibiotics, and safety policies, as well as education on such health hazards as tobacco, have led to drastic reductions in illnesses, including tuberculosis, diphtheria, pertussis, polio, hepatitis, lead poisoning, and cervical cancer. But the gain has not been distributed equally to all members of our society, and the causes of death have largely transformed from twentieth-century infectious threats to twenty-first-century chronic diseases. Repeating a similar success in the United States this century and extending life expectancy to 150 years by the year 2250 requires addressing disparities and altering personal behaviors amenable to change—both major tasks. Average life expectancy in the United States is currently 79 years, but it varies by up to 20 years among ethnic and geographic subpopulations.[2] Health disparities and a widening gap exist, with a 12-year difference in life expectancy between white females and African American males, and the average life expectancy ranging from 67 years in Oglala Lakota County, South Dakota, to 87 years in Summit County, Colorado. Global life expectancy also varies greatly, from over 90 years for females living in Monaco to less than 40 years for males born in Angola.

The World Health Organization (WHO) estimates that by 2020 two-thirds of all causes of death worldwide will be the result of lifestyle choices. Heart disease and cancer currently account for 50 percent of all deaths in the United States, and chronic disease is the major cause of disability.[3] Living longer creates a paradox, requiring all of us to take better care of ourselves over longer periods. Addressing threats to health and promoting healthy habits such as an active lifestyle, healthy diet, and routine sleep are vital. Modifying high-risk behaviors, including through cessation of smoking, reduction of substance abuse, use of safe-sex practices, and management of chronic stress, is critical. While changing behaviors is not easy, strategies and resources to improve the health of the population must be a priority.

A healthy health-care workforce is more important now than ever before. Physicians and other health professionals have the knowledge and skills to motivate patients to implement effective strategies to stop smoking, eat a healthy diet, maintain regular exercise, moderate alcohol use, manage stress, and maintain adequate sleep. But they are also at great risk and must be trained and supported if they are expected to model and sustain their own health.

## Defining Health and Wellness

Health defined broadly is synonymous with wellness and well-being. This biopsychosocial model of health has replaced the traditional biologic model.

The World Health Organization, in its 1946 constitution, defined *health* as a "state of complete physical, mental, and social well-being and not merely the absence of disease."[4] *Wellness*, according to the World Health Organization, "refers to diverse and interconnected dimensions of physical, mental, and social well-being that extend beyond the traditional definition of health. It encompasses choices and activities aimed at achieving physical vitality, mental alacrity, social satisfaction, a sense of accomplishment, and personal fulfillment."[4,5] The Vanderbilt University Wellness Wheel depicts health comprehensively within seven dimensions: physical, spiritual, social, intellectual, occupational, environmental, and emotional. Each of these areas is vital to understanding threats to wellness that affect us; all areas are interconnected, uniquely at risk in the twenty-first century, and can be improved though actionable strategies.

*Physical health* is the capability of our bodies to perform optimally. The top ten causes of death, including cardiovascular disease and cancer, are largely due to preventable behaviors, such as a sedentary lifestyle, poor diet, and tobacco use. Obesity is a growing epidemic, and tobacco is viewed as public health enemy number one, responsible for half of all cancers and over 70 percent of all deaths.[3] Adherence to evidence-based health guidelines, as written by the U.S. Preventive Services Task Force on topics including eating, sleeping, exercising, and using alcohol in moderation, can have a major impact on physical health, but overall adherence to many of these lifestyle recommendations falls below 10 percent.[6,3]

*Spiritual health* is the perception that life has meaning and purpose. While no specific religion has been shown to be superior in support of health, a commitment to self and others provides a shield against stress and adversity and promotes resilience to overcome major physical, emotional, and psychological trauma.[7] Spirituality and religion are protective in preventing and treating depression.[8] As a whole, our nation is becoming less religious, and we are at risk for perceiving less meaning in life. The Religious Landscape Study found a growing population of nonreligious Americans, up from 16 percent in 2007 to 23 percent in 2014. This absence of religious belief is particularly high in the millennial generation.[9]

*Social health* is a valuing of self as a member of an interconnected society. Strong relationships are consistently linked with wellness and are as important to health as diet and exercise. A full 40 percent of Americans reported "feeling lonely" in 2014.[10] Social isolation has been associated with major health consequences, including increased stress, lower immune responses, high blood pressure, and premature death; these were worse depending on the length and the severity of loneliness.[11-13] Connectivity in our highly plugged-in and fast-paced society presents new risks for isolation, particularly for teens.[14,15]

*Intellectual health* is the ability to achieve mastery and advancement through pursuit of educational interests, passions, and experiences. Education is one of the strongest contributors to social and economic status and health.[16] Exposure to new experiences and quality mentors stimulates inquiry and curiosity. Many people in the United States do not have access to or choices for quality education. Literacy and educational disparities limit opportunities for many and contribute to a spiral of poor health.

*Occupational health* is the satisfaction, outlook, and financial stability of professional work and a career. Dissatisfaction with work can lead to burnout and can have a negative impact on health. Satisfaction with work-life balance in the general population has increased from 55 percent to 61 percent between 2011 and 2014. Physicians' satisfaction with work-life balance in the same three years has declined from 49 percent to 41 percent.[17] Facets of work that contribute to dissatisfaction and burnout include a perceived excessive workload; lack of autonomy, recognition, sense of community, and trust; and poor alignment of personal to organizational values.[18] Work settings that uphold a high moral standard, set clear expectations, align vision to values, and support personal development can positively contribute to an individual's health. Those that do not can be toxic and can destroy our well-being.

*Environmental health* is the capacity to benefit from the conditions within which one works, plays, and lives. Clean air, water, shelter, and safe foods are basic survival needs. Exposure to the natural environment is also vital to health.[19] A supportive home, school, and work environment contributes to one's learning, personal growth, engagement, satisfaction, ability to contribute, and well-being. Health inequities and disparities exist among individuals who do not have access to or opportunities to live in safe and supportive environments. Adverse childhood experiences, such as abuse and neglect, lead to high-risk health behaviors, such as multiple sexual contacts and substance abuse, which in turn lead to chronic disease and increased mortality.[20]

*Emotional health* is the ability to cope with stress in a manner that maintains a positive mood and sense of self. While acute stress is protective, chronic stress is destructive. Chronic stress in the form of day-to-day overload is experienced as agitation, apprehension, fear, and anxiety. Over time it may lead to chronic fatigue, disengagement, distrust, burnout, and, for many, depression. The Harvard researchers Robert M. Yerkes and John D. Dodson in 1908 described how heightened arousal from stress increases performance up to a critical threshold, at which point it begins to have a negative effect.[21] Mental-health disorders are experienced by one in four Americans every year. The resulting demands on the health system are compounded by a shortage of mental-health–care providers.

## The Cause and Effect of Burnout

Chronic stress is a universal risk in today's frenetic society. Our can-do and must-do culture creates constant demands and places greater expectations and value on performance and achievement than on enjoyment, appreciation, and well-being. The culture of excess limits time for reflection and appreciation and leaves many harboring overwhelming feelings of negativity and hopelessness. Stress will soon replace tobacco as public health enemy number one, as it negatively affects all aspects of health, contributes to the incidence of chronic diseases such as anxiety and depression, and is a major factor in substance abuse, suicide, and the growing epidemic of burnout.

Burnout, which affects one in three working Americans and one in two health professionals, is defined as a "response to chronic stressors that wear on a person over time—not acute ones such as a big event or a big change" and as a "state of emotional exhaustion, depersonalization, cynicism and hostility, poor self-esteem and lack of empathy for others."[17,22] Burnout is a "progressive loss of idealism, energy, and purpose, experienced by people, particularly those in the helping professions, as a result of the conditions of their work."[23]

Burnout can mimic many physical or emotional health conditions, disguising itself as viral illness, weight changes, addiction, insomnia, agitation, hypertension, fatigue, and depression. Those experiencing burnout can present with frustration, cynicism, hostility, disengagement, distrust, and absence from work. Family members or colleagues may notice changes in motivation, satisfaction, or performance at home or at work. They may report, "She just stopped caring" or "He disengaged from everyone and everything." Many people with burnout experience isolation, which further aggravates the problem and contributes to a lack of self-confidence and a poor self-image.

Burnout is a serious concern for everyone, but it is found most frequently, and increasingly, in health professionals. In the United States 28 percent of the working population reported burnout in 2011, with no change in 2014. In the same three-year period the rates seen in our nation's physicians increased from 46 percent to an astounding 54 percent.[17] Burnout surfaces early in medical training and can be present throughout the careers of all health professionals; the rates of burnout among students, residents, physicians, nurses, and medical researchers all exceed 50 percent.[17,24-29]

Education promotes health and protects against burnout; given this fact, one would expect health professionals to have immunity. Recent data demonstrate the opposite. Compared to high school graduates, those with undergraduate and master's degrees experience a reduced likelihood of burnout, by 20 percent and 30 percent respectively. Doctoral degrees were associated with a nearly 40 percent reduction in burnout. The MD degree, however, was associated with a 40 percent increase. Rates of burnout in health professionals vary by gender, career stage, discipline, practice setting, and specialty, but no one in health care is immune.[17,30]

The number of physicians suffering from burnout, excluding nurses or other health professionals critical to the workforce, exceeds half a million (more than 40,000 medical students, 60,000 residents, and 490,000 physicians) and represents a public health crisis.[17,24] Despite training and expertise in screening patients for emotional and mental-health issues, health professionals are not reliable in assessing distress in themselves.[26,31]

The impact of burnout among health-care providers is felt by the providers themselves, the systems they work in, and society as a whole. Providers experiencing burnout have lower job satisfaction and increased rates of interpersonal conflict, substance use, depression, and suicide.[32-34] Medical students' depression rates have been reported as high as 55 percent, with an average of 27 percent, and suicidal ideation as high as 24 percent, with an average of 11 percent.[25,35] Health-care systems are negatively affected by increased costs and reduced productivity from job turnover, absenteeism, presenteeism, and early retirement.[36-39] Burnout in health-care providers has a magnified impact on the health of society, as it is associated with increased medical errors, poor quality of care, negative patient outcomes, and diminished patient satisfaction.[30,40-48]

Causes of burnout can be viewed from the same three perspectives: providers themselves, the systems they work in, and society as a whole. Society has and continues to hold physicians to higher expectations and unrealistic standards, contributing to an image of invincibility. Homer, the legendary Greek author of the *Iliad* and the *Odyssey*, claimed, "Society expects more of physicians because of their training."[49] Health professionals are expected to walk the walk, but this is not always easy or possible given the complex and demanding culture of medicine and medical education. Medicine, while profoundly rewarding, is one of the only professions in America in which the health and safety of their personnel is not top priority.

Medical and health-care systems continue to recognize and reward academic achievement and clinical productivity above all else. Individuals face diminished resources, expanded expectations, and a lack of balanced role models. Self-care strategies have not traditionally been included in medical education, nor are they assessed in performance metrics. Medicine and the health-care system are classically perceived by those experiencing burnout as having an excessive workload, administrative inefficiencies, and an overwhelming pace of organizational change.[17,46,50]

Toxicity begins early on. Upon entrance to medical school, students actually report better overall quality of life, as well as higher mental, physical, and emotional health and lower rates of burnout and depression than age-similar college graduates.[51] But this rapidly changes, and burnout is present in over half of first-year medical students, a rate similar to all health professionals and 20 percent above the general population. Depression rates in first-year medical students also jump to 30 percent, compared to 5 percent in their age-matched peers.[17] Those entering the profession are often high achievers and quickly adapt to the tradition seeped in perfectionism, hierarchy, self-sacrifice, guilt, and delayed gratification. The stigmas of self-care and mental health that exist within the general public are exaggerated among health professionals when they consider their own health. Traditional physician training and job descriptions have never included being healthy, and many health professionals interpret focusing on their own health needs as selfish, lazy, or weak. Health professionals are charged with achieving the triple aim: better health, better care, and lower costs for patients and for the health-care system. Aspiring academicians also answer to the quadruple threat: conducting research, educating future doctors, delivering clinical care, and leading teams. Motivated and naive students, who prior to medical school knew only success in all dimensions of health and life, should ask the realistic question: "Can I do all that and still be healthy myself?"

## *Medice Cura Te Ipsum*: Physician, Heal Thyself!

The Hippocratic Oath, written in Greek in the late fifth century BCE by Hippocrates, "the father of medicine," is still taken by every medical student upon graduation and includes the promise "to abstain from doing harm." This oath is a mandate to weigh the benefit and risk of all choices made on behalf of our patients, and this includes the impact of our own health, or lack thereof, on the health of those for whom we provide care. To avert the declining wellness of health professionals and to overcome the existing gaps in national health outcomes, we as health professionals must change our culture, and this means we must first and foremost prioritize our own wellness, just as we expect our patients to do—no more, no less.

Medicine remains one of the noblest of all vocations, but it is embedded in a tradition of relentless demands and self-sacrifice. Personal health has long been a missing component in the culture of medicine, and this has major consequences for the health of the general population. This problem is growing despite advances in technology and innovation, and it demands the collective efforts of society, health systems, and professionals to solve.

In 2014 Drs. Thomas Bodenheimer and Christine Sinsky addressed the epidemic by challenging the traditional triple aim and proposing the quadruple aim: "Health care providers can't achieve the Triple Aim's core ideals without first prioritizing their own health needs."[52] Understanding factors that threaten well-being is necessary to design effective solutions. Individual and system-wide, evidence-based wellness initiatives are emerging, but quality research demonstrating sustainable impact is still limited.[25,30,40,53-56]

Interventions aimed at individuals can also be used by organizations, as leaders within organizations must change for systems to change, and systems-based changes are needed to support individual change. The power to improve the populations health lies within each individual's capacity to advance self-care.

To improve our nation's health, we as medical professionals must model self-care. To overcome the epidemic of burnout that has disproportionally hit our profession and be accountable to the public, we must be accountable to ourselves. Doing so positively affects our own health, permits others to do the same, and transforms medical culture to improve the health of teams, organizations, communities, and ultimately the entire population. Promoting the health of society takes a community and requires a change of systems, but ultimately it is the individual who has the responsibility and the power to promote personal wellness.

# PART ONE SELF-AWARENESS

• ✦ ● ▶ ✦ ● ● ● ✦ ▸ ▪

The unexamined life is not worth living.

SOCRATES

Self-awareness sets the stage for self-discovery and continuous personal growth and development. This takes time, requires practice, and is never finished. Knowledge of one's current state of wellness and potential health challenges can empower self-care and self-improvements. Awareness begins with observation, includes inquiry and self-assessment, and concludes with a commitment to ongoing reflection to sustain understanding of oneself.

• ◦ ● ● ► ● ● ● ● ● ◦ ►

# BE PRESENT

*Yesterday is history, tomorrow is mystery, today is a gift.*
ELEANOR ROOSEVELT

When I first met Hannah, an admired vice president at a community hospital, she was forty and described her previous self as a "numbers" person. She had found purpose in achievements and accomplishments that could be counted on her résumé. She had children when she was young, then returned to school, determined to have a meaningful career. Hannah came to me to establish primary care at the advice of her oncologist. She had recently returned from visiting her three children, who were all away at college. When her children had left the previous fall, she had been too busy to take time off and take them to their schools. But now, after being diagnosed with breast cancer, she rented a house near their different colleges, cooked their favorite meals, met their professors, visited with their friends, and engaged in their lives. She brought photographs and shared stories of their childhoods in an attempt to immortalize memories. She told them she loved them and how lucky she felt to be their mother, and she shared her new mantra: "Cherish each *day* as if it is your last." She also advised them to be tested for the BRCA1 gene, which she carried but hoped she hadn't shared with them.

Five years later, at forty-five, Hannah was free of cancer and considered cured. Reflecting back over the course of her life and her courses of chemotherapy, Hannah acknowledged that her life had changed suddenly with her diagnosis. She had always been driven, but without direction. But when she thought she was dying, she felt more alive. She spoke of the highs and lows and her awe at the reality of seeing an end to life. It forced her to stop and look at herself and all that was around her. She observed a wide range of feelings: denial, exhaustion, sadness, curiosity, fear, grief, and joy. Her head had grown shiny, no longer bouncing with dark curls, and her skin had thinned: side effects of the chemotherapy. Friends and colleagues worldwide wrote to her, and she shared with me her stamp collection from around the globe. No longer working her sixty-plus hours a week, she began to focus on art, a passion she had given up for her career as an administrator in health care. The range of colors and the texture and smell of her paintings now filled her world. And despite knowing she was cured, Hannah remained committed to feeling fully alive every day.

Four years after Hannah celebrated her cure, I was paged by Radiology. "I've never seen such rapid progression of disease," my colleague said, while reviewing Hannah's routine annual scan. She agreed to keep Hannah at Radiology until I arrived. Hannah wept calmly when she saw me, her dark curls once again bouncing, as she sat alone in the small radiology suite. Her husband was working, fully expecting to hear about a negative scan when they talked later.

She whispered that she had experienced nausea and stomach pain most of the summer, but since her children were home, she chose to focus on them. Her screenings over the past four years had all been normal, and so she thought she could wait. Her scan revealed widely metastatic disease with cancer spread to her liver, lungs, and bowels. Later that fall, in what would be her last office visit, she shared a new mantra: "Cherish each *moment* as if it is your last." She lived her life in a way that I wasn't sure I could. She was not naive; she knew that being present in each moment would not cure her cancer, but she was grateful it had freed her to focus on what mattered—her health and her family.

Eight weeks later I visited Hannah in the hospital while she received experimental chemotherapy. Standard treatments had not worked. Christmas carolers passed from one section of the infusion suite to the next; Hannah's family sang along. I knew each of them, as Hannah had set up her children and husband with appointments to ensure that their health needs were addressed and they were cared for in her absence. I held back my tears, fearful of their effect on her. Being in Hannah's presence alerted my senses: I saw her shiny head, once again lacking those dark bouncy curls; heard the words of

"Silent Night"; smelled hospital care; and touched the thinning smooth skin of a peacefully dying woman. When the song ended, I asked, "How are you?"

She turned from the carolers, giving me her full attention. "I am wonderful. Aren't they lovely? How are your girls? What are your holiday plans?"

I shared minimally, again fearful of sparking memories of dreams she dared not dream. "Is there anything I can do for you?" I asked.

"Nothing at all. I have no pain, no worries, no bucket list, haven't had one for years." She went on without prompting. "My family is all set. We've said all that needs saying and done all that we could do. Everything I need is right here." She shared how she agreed with Lou Gehrig, who, knowing he was to die and having had time to say good-bye, said in his farewell speech, "Today, I consider myself the luckiest man on the face of the earth."[57] Hannah told me how lucky she felt to know me and thanked me for everything. She pushed me to say good-bye, to go home to my family, and then she hugged me for the last time. I watched Hannah and her husband and three children singing joyously as I left the unit.

I never saw Hannah again. She died on December 15, my birthday.

Hannah was one of my many patients with cancer, and while she did not live any longer than others, she was unique in her acceptance of both her life and her death. During the nine years I cared for her, she shared that it was the cancer that made her mindful and taught her and her family to focus on what mattered. She was truly grateful for the opportunity to fully live as she was dying.

## Mindfulness

Mindfulness has been defined as people's "ability to be purposefully and non-judgmentally attentive to their own experience, thoughts and feelings."[58] Jon Kabat-Zinn, founding director of the Stress Reduction Clinic and the Center for Mindfulness in Medicine, Health Care, and Society at the University of Massachusetts Medical School, describes it as a "waking up and living in harmony with oneself and with the world."[59,157] Mindfulness is synonymous with meditation, which has philosophical and spiritual roots dating to before Christ, before Buddha, and even before Aristotle.

Numerous tools have been developed to measure mindfulness. One, the

Mindful Attention Awareness Scale (MAAS), was created to capture attention and awareness in daily life. It contains fourteen items on a six-point Likert scale and is used around the world, having been translated into many languages.[60] The questions reflect one's attention and focus in the moment, asking, for example, if you find yourself "listening to someone with one ear, doing something else at the same time.[53] The higher the MAAS score, the more the perceived level of mindfulness.

Over the past five years there has been a growing body of literature on the broad advantages and health benefits of mindfulness to physical, spiritual, social, intellectual, occupational, and emotional well-being. Publications on mindfulness have risen from 52 in 2003 to 477 in 2012, with nearly 100 randomized, controlled trials published by 2014.[61] In addition to reduced stress, diminished disease burden, and increased job satisfaction for those practicing mindfulness, benefits extend beyond the individual to others; in the case of health-care providers, benefits extend to their patients.

REDUCED STRESS AND THE BURDEN OF DISEASE    The practice of mindfulness is a potent remedy to counter the physiological effects of acute and chronic stress and is comparable to other strategies that have proven effective, including cognitive behavioral therapy (CBT) and medication.[62-64] Mindfulness fosters a natural state of equilibrium within us and with the world around us. Reported benefits of mindfulness include enhanced focus, relaxation, compassion, acceptance, productivity, peace, and happiness, along with diminished agitation, avoidance, fatigue, anxiety, and burnout.[65,66]

Being mindful reduces the effects of illness in patients who have pain and provides benefits in a range of other health conditions. While there is no evidence that mindfulness prevents or cures disease, extensive studies and randomized controlled trials demonstrate its effectiveness in symptom relief, improved quality of life, and stress reduction.[67,68] Measurable biochemical changes in immune function, levels of cortisol, dehydroepiandrosterone sulfate, (DHEA-S), and melatonin as well as reduced pain and stress have been shown with mindfulness practice in patients with cancer, psoriasis, eating disorders, anxiety, and depression.[69-73] In a controlled study of cancer patients, higher MAAS scores were associated with lower mood disturbance and lower stress symptoms.[60] Elderly patients who adopted mindfulness practices lived longer than elderly patients who did not.[74] Ongoing studies show promising results in the use of mindfulness to manage fibromyalgia and to treat substance abuse.[75-77]

INCREASED JOB PERFORMANCE    Mindful reflection that occurs before and after work activities provides valuable feedback and increases work effectiveness. In *The Power of Mindful Learning*, Dr. Ellen J. Langer, a professor of psychology at Harvard, reported that a "mindful approach to any activity has three characteristics: the continuous creation of new categories, openness to new information, and an implicit awareness of more than one perspective."[74] Benefits go beyond the individual to the system. Organizations that incorporate mindful reflection into daily work find that employees understand successes and failures, perform better, and are rejuvenated in ways that are similar to their taking short breaks or vacations.[50]

IMPACTS FOR HEALTH-CARE PROVIDERS AND THEIR PATIENTS    Just as burnout in health-care providers negatively affects providers and patients, mindfulness training of medical students, residents, nurses, and physicians has been shown to improve their personal well-being, patient-care skills, and clinical competence.[46,58,78,79] The goal of mindfulness in medicine is to increase inner awareness of caregivers' mental processes and to promote their active listening.[58] In a 2013 multicenter study, physicians' self-ratings of mindfulness using the MAAS were compared to audio recordings of their patient visits. Higher self-scores were associated with greater patient satisfaction and higher-quality patient care, which was determined by longer visits, greater efficiency, enhanced communication and empathy, greater listening skills, a higher degree of reported trust, and stronger patient-doctor relationships.[80] Providers trained in mindfulness techniques for as little as two and a half hours per week for eight weeks have had increased patient and provider satisfaction. Providers with improved mindfulness report reduced burnout; reduced emotional exhaustion and depersonalization; and improved mood, personal well-being, sense of accomplishment, and empathy to their patients' emotional and social lives.[58,78,79]

## Learning to Be Mindful

Like Hannah, I used to race from one task to another, proudly multitasking along the way; the concept of focusing on one thing was foreign to me. I first discovered the benefits of mindfulness in a yoga class I took prior to attending medical school. The class began and ended with guided reflection. Simple calming words directed my attention away from work, away from future plans, and toward the present moment. Previously, I had exercised mindlessly amid my flurry of thoughts, oblivious to the exercise experience. I would run in DC and miss the Washington Monument, run along the Maine coast and miss even the ocean. Missing experiences was not limited to exercise. I would eat and not remember what I had eaten or even that I had eaten. Paradoxically, yoga felt like a minibreak from life; actually, I became more present in the now. Practicing yoga was the first time I felt diverted away from the undone and the to-do. Being in the present for a class, I observed my feelings transform from overload to calm, "like the surface of the lake," as the instructor suggested. I was stunned at how grounded and renewed I felt after a brief sixty minutes. I was equally amazed at how fast the calmness left me when I exited the studio and returned to my life. I began practicing meditative yoga for ten minutes at the beginning and end of each day, hoping that the more I practiced, the more I would feel replenished.

As a medical student, I found myself overloaded, and I felt pressure to do even more, guilt if I missed an opportunity, and fear of the smallest failure. I went from classes to the library to the hospital, always believing I needed to be elsewhere. My mind raced, my fear grew, and I became stuck and began worrying, getting little accomplished and feeling fearful I would let others down. I lost focus and appreciation for what previously had mattered. There was not enough time in the day to exercise, cook, take photos, read (anything other than anatomy), socialize, or even sleep or eat well. Life was a battle, and I was losing. Past skills were no longer strengths. I no longer organized my time. I was afraid to acknowledge even silently to myself that my pace was not sustainable. I experienced no pleasure from what had previously brought me joy, and I was often too busy for my ten-minute minibreaks. It was my mother who pointed out the obvious. "You are not happy," she observed. "Is medicine really what you want to do?"

Awareness of the moment guided me when my brother shared a copy of *The Pocket Thich Nhất Hạnh*. This miniature version of the story of a Buddhist monk, exiled from Vietnam for his political message on peace, equates mindfulness with peace, suggesting it exists only in the present moment. I felt Nhất Hạnh describe my life when he wrote about the hope of peace. "It is ridiculous to say, wait until I finish this, then I will be free to live in peace. What is this, a diploma, a job, a house, the payment of a debt? If you think that way, peace will never come. There is always another 'this' that will follow the present one. If you are not living in peace at this moment, you will never be able to. If you truly want to be at peace, you must be at peace right now. Otherwise, there is only 'the hope of peace someday.'"[81]

As I wondered how to stop waiting and to be at peace now, I reflected on the words of Dr. Benjamin Bacharach, dean of admissions, who had oriented me on my first day at Jefferson Medical College. "Don't let medicine be an excuse for not living," he said. But my mind was elsewhere, and only later did the words sink in. At the time I was thinking, *I shouldn't miss my nephew's christening; I should be there, but I need to be here studying. . . .* After reading and rereading *The Pocket Thich Nhất Hạnh*, which I kept in my white coat, I took the Day of Mindfulness challenge. I found Sundays, my chosen day, to be peaceful, replenishing, and surprisingly productive. I began using the yoga-based reflection before studying, and I felt the same intensity for physiology as for yoga. Addressing one task at a time, I again found joy in learning. The pressure and fear subsided. Since then I have assimilated mindfulness while running, cooking, walking in the woods with my husband, talking with my daughters, attending budget committees, facing fears, and listening to patients. Being in the moment changed my perception of mindfulness from a ten-minute exercise to a way of living.

During my fourth year of medical school, I completed an elective with the World Health Organization at Chulalongkorn University in Thailand. Our community project—teaching mothers to boil water for their newborn babies—seemed simple, but was not. The fact that I spoke only a few phrases of Thai forced me into perpetual mindfulness. With heightened senses I observed everything around me as I walked in Bangkok, attempted tai chi in Phuket, and dived into my pile of books. *Wherever You Go, There You Are: Mindfulness Meditation in Everyday Life*, by Jon Kabat-Zinn, reminded me that the grass is greener elsewhere only when we address the reason we're searching for greener pastures to begin with.[59] *The Miracle of Mindfulness: An Introduction to the Practice of Mindfulness*, by Thich Nhất Hạnh, expanded my scope of mindfulness to an "act of concentrated awareness and a keeping of one's consciousness alive to the present reality."[82]

Over the years I continued to practice mindfulness occasionally, the way most women report doing self–breast exams only when they consciously think about it. My life as a physician, mother, teacher, and wife often distracted me from being present now. Hannah retaught me. The greatest gift we have to give is our time and attention, and the time to be attentive is always now. When we devote time and attention to something or someone, including ourselves, we declare what matters to us. Constructing an efficient agenda at work gives colleagues the message that they matter. Sharing a leisurely meal with family implies that those relationships matter. Listening actively to patients' stories tells them they matter. Discussing children's fears in an unhurried manner tells them their emotions matter. Prioritizing self-care affirms for me that my health matters.

By being in the now, Hannah diminished past worries and future fears. Focusing in the moment simplified her life by freeing her senses to observe only current details. To focus is to limit distractions and attend to a priority fully. Hannah told me that she found moving mindlessly from one thing to another was draining her and preventing her from accomplishing anything well. When chronic overload becomes the norm, it blocks our attainment of health and happiness. Hannah stopped, observed her world, and brought unconscious thoughts and feelings to consciousness. She saw details she otherwise missed, particularly in everyday things: family, friends, her home, painting, nature, and herself. Driving to the beach, she smelled the ocean; savoring a bite of cake, she tasted the burst of dark chocolate; watching her child brush her teeth, she felt pride.

Other key aspects of a mindfulness practice are acceptance and the withholding of judgment in observing situations, people, perspectives, biases, and even prejudices. In *Zen Mind, Beginner's Mind: Informal Talks on Zen Meditation and Practice*, Shunryu Suzuki emphasizes this: "In the beginner's mind there are many possibilities, but in the expert's there are few."[83] He highlights the strengths of those coming to mindfulness from a place of "inquiry" and openness to learning. Acceptance, he writes, is the peace that comes with letting life happen—without forcing it. It is a belief in our interconnectedness with nature and the universe. Hannah accepted the natural process of life, just as farmers who raise animals accept death as part of life. She used the phrase "That's life" not as a sign of hopelessness but as a sign of letting go. Hannah made a conscious choice each day to act purposefully, and by devoting more time to fewer things, she fostered intense gratitude for what she had in the moment. Hannah modeled gratitude, and her family followed, refusing to wait and recognize their love for her only after losing her.

## Barriers to Mindfulness

Being mindful is harder than one might think. In *Wherever You Go, There You Are*, Jon Kabat-Zinn describes how mindfulness is "simple, but not easy."[59] Obstacles to mindfulness can be cultural and personal. Hannah and I both experienced the fast-paced, multitasking culture of both medicine and the American lifestyle. The value society places on doing more is a threat to being in the moment. Mindfulness is not about *doing* more but about *being* who you already are.

Multitasking is the opposite of mindfulness. Despite the movement of Western culture and medicine to embrace mindfulness, multitasking re-mains extrinsically rewarded. Like many colleagues, I have proudly mastered multitasking in my personal and professional life. Aided by technology and a plugged-in culture, I write notes, respond to texts, clear emails, and empty my patient task bin, all while simultaneously answering a colleague's question. I miss hearing what matters to a patient when my mind wanders to undone charts, other tasks, or other patients. Patients do the same: answering my question, disciplining their children, glancing at buzzing phones, and concur-rently showing me their erupting rash. When I catch my thoughts wandering and redirect them back to the patient without judging, I can focus completely on that person, which is powerful.

Rushing was another obstacle to Hannah's smelling the roses. She often found herself saying, "Let me just get *this* over with, just get my work done, just hurry and eat, just finish my calls." This mentality focuses on quantity and not quality, but it is the mainstay of many activities on many days for many people. Limiting what we do allows for a pace that feels doable. Setting boundaries provides more pleasure and less stress; it reduces the distressing feeling of never being where you want to be, never doing what you want to do, and never being done. Hannah, a self-described workaholic, found that being in the moment meant that things are dealt with when they arise. Something either mattered and got done, or it didn't matter. She came to see being mindful as a critical part of her performance at home and at work.

The presence of unexamined biases, beliefs, and past experiences also blocks the ability to be present.[83] A beginner might think or say, "I can't do this; I will never be able to meditate," or "Reflection is doing nothing, and action is what matters" or "I am too busy for this." Perfectionists desire to do it perfectly and focus on acquiring theory instead of consciousness. Both approaches result in self-judgment and perceived failure. A practiced meditator might say, "Reflection allows me time for creativity and space for learning," or "Observing gives me new insights and ideas and makes me more efficient and ultimately saves time." Beginners who keep an open mind and consciously reframe their thoughts have the ability to choose to react differently. Consciously observing one's thoughts provides access to overcoming barriers. Being mindful requires only observing thoughts and noting them. Changing thoughts is another strategy, which will be expanded on in lesson 11. Additional barriers to mindfulness in health professionals include a personal fear of self-absorption and lack of training.[58] Mindfulness can be viewed as a tool, just as the stethoscope is a tool, for promoting effective patient care; competence requires practice.

## The Practice of Mindfulness

Mindfulness research, training, and practice have surged in popularity in the twenty-first century. Practicing mindfulness comes from within; I don't need to go elsewhere to find it. It is in me—a feeling of being free, free to live in the space between past and future; free from fear, guilt, and judgment; free to blossom and do what I do best. Refusing to multitask or mindlessly do more provides time to be mindful. Stephen Covey, an expert on leadership, states, "The key is not to prioritize what's on your schedule, but to schedule your priorities."[84] Mindfulness requires time and prioritization. Scheduling time for mindfulness is a declaration that it matters, and practicing it daily for at least twenty-one days will ingrain it as a life habit. Thankfully, the act of being mindful does not require a terminal diagnosis; it can be achieved by paying attention to triggers, such as our own breath, body sensations, feelings, thoughts, or actions, or by simply observing others and our interactions in the world. Different triggers occur for different people at different times and in different situations.

Teaching mindfulness is a bit paradoxical. It can't be taught with traditional methods used for biology or anatomy. Learners must experience it; experts serve not as teachers but as guides or role models. The master multitasking medical student asks, "How can I be mindful?" My response is based on my own continuous effort, which always needs practice. I highlight children as our best role models. Children evoke the "hurry up" response from adults as they stop to smell the roses, listen to a fire truck, feel a grain of sand, taste cookie batter, and see the intricate patterns of snowflakes. Nothing is too mundane for a child's curiosity. Mindfulness is a skill we are born with, but, like muscle mass, it atrophies with disuse. We lose it when we race through the present, worry about the past, and fear the future. Simply refocusing on the current moment permits us to recapture our childlike appreciation of the world around us. Mindfulness requires practice, but in this case practice does not make perfect. The practice is the reward itself. In the words of the Zen master Shunryu Suzuki, "the practice of becoming a Zen is the enlightenment itself." He said, "When you eat, eat! Taste your food. Be in the moment. Be yourself. Just be present. That is the practice."[83]

In the classroom and in the office, mindfulness is a powerful tool for promoting self-awareness and focus. I try to model it as I first experienced it in yoga class. My goal is to foster participants' focus on a topic, no matter what the subject: diabetes, public health, team development, or personal health improvement. I ask learners and patients if they have ever meditated or practiced mindfulness. Surprised at the growing numbers, I proceed to invite all to "be with me in this moment, unplug from electronics, set aside thoughts of unfinished work and future 'to-do' lists." I ask all to "focus on now and notice their breath, feelings, and thoughts." I frame mindfulness as a first step toward slowing the pace, to see and understand one's health, life, and world. I demonstrate brief mindfulness exercises and provide opportunities for students to apply them personally. Participants express universal appreciation for focusing mindfully. A resident who completed Jon Kabat-Zinn's two-minute raisin exercise, where one devotes a powerful 120 seconds to feeling, seeing, smelling, tasting, and swallowing a single small piece of dried fruit, stated, "that was the first thing I tasted all month." A nurse shared regretfully that "I focused more on the raisin than I have on my child recently." A medical student shared, "I appreciate this permission coming from the top down and being lived out by faculty." I recommend Kabat-Zinn's readings to patients and mentees who wish to slow down their pace, value their health, and enjoy their lives.

In 2015 I had the opportunity to teach in China, one of the homes of Eastern medicine and meditation. In China the mindful walk is slower, the practice more purposeful, and the message more public. Confucianism still permeates the culture, and there is pride in the belief that others benefit from our mindfulness. While there, I read *Confucius Lives Next Door*, by T. R. Reid, and was reminded that individual responsibility for meditation is a means to promote personal balance as well as societal harmony.[85] Walking on the Great Wall of China, I was mindful of my and others' experience when multitasking to capture a photo on my phone.

After my China experience, while rushing to work one morning, I noticed mind*less*ness seeping back into my life. I had a long to-do list at my desk and was already running late when I encountered construction and came to a full stop on the highway. Having grown up hating the traffic in New Jersey, I expected my instinctual feelings of frustration, agitation, and internal shouting: *I have important things to do; I can't wait.* But that morning, sitting in traffic, it was as if Hannah or Confucius were in the car coaching me. I observed an intense feeling of appreciation and a new flow of thoughts; it's great to have extra minutes to focus on my breath before work. This transition from agitation to acceptance and appreciation was foreign, but persisted and affected my interactions with others in the office, in my patient's room, and in my home. What seemed like minor construction that morning gave me great pause that evening, as my acceptance seemed contagious. I, in turn, reaped the benefits of others' being less stressed. I was rewarded, not externally with accomplishments or titles, but internally with balance and happiness.

Remembering Hannah and her family inspires me. Her breast cancer, with all its pain and stresses, reminded her every day of all that she had. Complications and side effects of treatment that had the potential to extend suffering and negatively affect her care by increasing pain, lessening appetite, and disrupting sleep and relationships actually served as triggers for her being present and appreciating her life. She cared for her physical, emotional, and social health better with her terminal illness than she had prior to it. Physicians cannot predict how patients will respond to illness physiologically or psychologically, but we do know that those who live mindfully, as Hannah did, have less suffering and experience higher-quality lives.[86,87] As I reflect on Hannah's journey and her ability to reframe her health, I see a wise young woman with bouncy dark curls who taught me not to wait for greener pastures but to appreciate now. Nathaniel Hawthorne describes this experience as the "perfect future in the present."[88]

. . . . . . . . . . . .

HEALTH CHALLENGE #1   Practice Mindfulness

Do not look back on happiness or dream of it in the future.
You are only sure of today; do not let yourself be cheated out of it.
HENRY WARD BEECHER

Give yourself the gift of mindfulness by devoting ten minutes a day for the next thirty days to the practice. Declare this time important by placing it on your calendar. Use the MAAS tool prior to and after thirty days to assess changes in your level of mindfulness over time. Identify any of the following triggers to begin or advance your mindfulness journey. Complete the practice over and over, gradually extending your practice to an hour, a day, a week, and a lifetime.

1. Focus on your breath: Notice the inhalation and the exhalation. Listen to the breath and observe the length of inhalation and exhalation without trying to change the pattern. Count ten breaths or focus for ten minutes to start.

2. Scan your physical body: Bring awareness of sensation from toe to head. While lying down, sitting in a plane, standing, or hiking a

mountain, begin to tighten and relax each muscle group as you move from your feet up to your scalp. Be conscious of the tendency to view your experience as good or bad. Sensations are not to be judged, only perceived.

3. Appreciate your emotions: Consciously ask yourself, What am I feeling? Is there a predominant mood, or are there mixed emotions? Am I tense? Happy? Sad? Apprehensive? Excited? Disappointed? This can feel awkward, and there may be a tendency to label feelings as good or bad, or to deny or dwell on uncomfortable feelings. Observe and record feelings without assessing their value. Appreciate that we are wired to experience a full spectrum of emotions and that doing so is okay, even if the emotion is "hopeless."

4. Examine your thoughts: Consciously note the internal statements you are making about your breath, body, emotion, or other experience. Ask yourself, "What is my voice repeating regarding this sensation, feeling, or situation?" Listen openly without judgment. Thoughts can turn to beliefs and personal truths. Thoughts can have great impact on our behaviors, and while limiting thoughts can imprison us, positive thoughts can empower us. "This is going to be a great/horrible day!" "I can/can't do anything!" Observe how your thoughts are a replay of past experiences and how they are brought to the present and move with you to the future.

5. Focus attention outside yourself: Give your full attention to a single person, place, or thing, as if you have never seen it before. Complete Jon Kabat-Zinn's raisin exercise. And then consider a similar experience with your spouse or a child, pet, flower, food, friend, or colleague. Note any thoughts or judgments as you concentrate entirely outside yourself. Envision your part in the larger interconnected world. Consider how you interact with others. Observe the effects of your thoughts, feelings, and actions on others, and theirs on you.

• • • • • • • • • • • • •

# ASK QUESTIONS

A prudent question is one half of wisdom.

SIR FRANCIS BACON

## First Visit

Carmen was scheduled at three o'clock for a new-patient physical exam. This new-patient, "get to know you" visit miraculously means I get to spend an hour with the patient. My nurse, Deb, diligently screened the sixty-year-old female for past preventive services and noted gaps in documenting mammograms and pap smears. She inquired about accessing past records. Deb prepared the room, placed the speculum on the tray, printed ID labels for the cervical specimen, and added lab requests to the electronic chart. Deb summarized Carmen by saying she had recently moved to the area, was here to establish care, and had no specific questions or concerns.

When I entered the room, Carmen was visibly nervous, looking sideways from the corner of her eyes and moving her fingers in circles on her lap. I reached out to shake her hand; she stood, reserved and cautious, and reached back. I began, as with all new encounters, by saying, "I'm Dr. Pipas. It is a pleasure to meet you. Welcome. Please tell me about yourself."

She responded to me with a question: "Will you be my primary-care physician?" Her fingers continued to circle, flipping over a half-size yellow notepad, revealing a short list printed neatly in tiny block lettering. She quietly informed me that she would not need a pap smear, as she did not have a uterus. I nodded, as this is often the case in postmenopausal women who have had a hysterectomy. She proceeded to ask me again, "Are you willing to take me on as a patient," adding softly, "given I was previously a 'he'?"

I looked at her for what must have seemed like forever, looking for signs of what I had not previously noticed. She was tall, over five feet ten, well over two hundred pounds; her brownish-grayish hair was thinning and pulled tightly into a bun; and her face was tan, with a hint of foundation lighter than the surrounding areas. Her skin was smooth, with gentle signs of aging, making her appear younger than sixty. She wore blue dress slacks, pressed stiffly, with a striped mauve blouse and a blue cardigan sweater. A delicate gold cross hung around her neck and her penny loafers were well worn. No signs, I thought to myself, as I responded to her question: "To be honest, I don't know what your needs are—physically, mentally, emotionally, or sexually—but I am willing to learn." I asked her again to tell me about herself: who she was and what her goals were.

She smiled briefly and nodded, then she steadied her hands, scanned her notes, and began to speak. "I have diabetes, high blood pressure, depression, and hypothyroidism. I take Metformin, Enalopril, Paxil, Synthroid, and Premarin." She went on with details of each illness, as many patients do, interpreting my broad inquiry to be about diseases. I learned about her chronic illnesses, her medication side effects, recent lab results, overdue lab tests, and medications that needed refills. But still I knew nothing about Carmen the person. Caring effectively for one sixty-year old patient with diabetes and depression is just that. Even if two patients have identical backgrounds, risks, and illnesses, their health-care needs differ. I wasn't sure how her gender transition would affect her health, but I was certain that being transgender wouldn't make her more or less like any other patient or more or less complex in her needs.

Being a physician is an honor and a learning experience, and caring for Carmen would be no exception. My learning curve, however, would be steeper than usual, not because she was transgender and not because she had *not* previously considered many of the questions I would ask of her, but because she would become such a willing teacher and I, new to the care of transgender patients, had much to learn. I knew that providing a safe space for inquiry without judgment would be critical. Given that my experience caring for transgender patients was nil, I had no box to put her in, and so I began with a clean slate. I was curious and assumed nothing, like the novice meditator and ancient philosopher who apologized to the scholar for not having the answer, saying, "I do not know what is right, but in not knowing I am open to learning more." For thousands of years teachers have described the power of a good question to aid in the learning process. As Voltaire directs, "judge a man by his questions rather than his answers."[89] The Socratic method establishes questions as valuable tools for critical thinking and fostering active learning in all settings. Teaching through questions is powerful in the office, in the classroom, and in life.

The root of "doctor," *docere*, comes from Latin and means "to teach." Ironically, most of my learning comes from those I teach. The more questions I ask, the more I learn; the more I learn, the better I am as a teacher. I support the notion that no question is a dumb question, and my learning is reciprocated when students and patients trust and contribute to open dialogue and question me. As a mother, I play the "what if" game, encouraging my daughters to explore the consequences of their choices. What if you eat chocolate before dinner? What if you don't wear a seat belt? What if you get in a car with someone who has been drinking? What if you allow someone to mistreat you? I continuously ask myself fundamental questions. Who am I? What matters to me? Am I balanced in my giving and taking?

Appreciative inquiry (AI) is a complementary and specific method of questioning that seeks to uncover the best in people, situations, or topics. Skilled leaders and facilitators use it to emphasize positive aspects of inquiry: What worked well in our project? What was the highlight of my day? What do you love about your spouse? AI is based on the principle that, although both good and bad occur in life constantly, if we choose to focus on the positive, we appreciate that which is going well. AI generates positive energy. I utilize AI with patients and students, sharing the legend of the Cherokee elder and his grandchildren that I was told as a child. The elder tells them, "In everyone's life there is a terrible fight—a fight between two wolves. One is evil: he is fear, anger, envy, greed, arrogance, self-pity, resentment, and deceit. The other is good: he is joy, serenity, humility, confidence, generosity, truth, gentleness, and compassion." One of the children asks, "Grandfather, which wolf will win?" The elder replies, "The one you feed."[90]

Over the course of the next hour, and the next six years, I would ask Carmen numerous positively framed questions. I reiterated that there were no right or wrong answers and no red pen to grade or judge her. I shared how those who had previously considered these fundamental questions might have quick answers, while others, to whom they might be new, would need time to explore and might find the questions uncomfortable or difficult to answer. I told Carmen it was okay if her reaction was any of these.

I began by inquiring about her general strengths and asked simple questions. "What do you do well?"

Carmen, hesitated, again her finger circling. "I don't know."

I listened and waited in silence, but nothing more came. I expanded my question: "What do others say you do well?"

She scratched notes on her pad but did not speak. She offered that she found it difficult to talk about herself, but that she could write down her thoughts.

"You are good at writing?" I prompted.

She offered that she kept lists.

"Perfect!" I concluded. "Can you make me a list of the things you do well? If it helps, you can start each item with 'I think I am good at . . .' or 'People say I am good at . . .'"

She offered that she would like to give it a try, but it might take her some time. We agreed that my nurse, Deb, would check on her, and that I would see my last patients and be back in thirty minutes. I also asked her to consider another question. "What goals do you have?"

A perplexed blank stare crossed her face.

I clarified. "What would you do if you had more hours in the day or days in the week?"

Her spinning fingers grasped the pen and left tiny marks on her yellow notepad. I left Carmen in the examining room to write. Two ear infections later I returned. She had a short list printed in tiny block letters. "How did you do"? I asked.

She looked up and smiled softly. Silence.

"Would you share your strengths with me?" I asked. She handed me the notepad, opened to a page titled "What Others Say about Me." I handed it back and asked her to read it to me. She read the list verbatim.

1. You are the best cook in the house.
2. You are an efficient and frugal grocery shopper.

3. You are a dependable, organized employee with good problem-solving skills.
4. You are a patient teacher and a strong coach and trainer of new employees.
5. You are soft.

"Sounds like others see you as an asset at home and at work?"

She nodded.

"What does it mean and who describes you as soft?" I inquired.

Silence. She glanced down and turned the page over. I could see a second list on the next page. Silence. She jokingly answered my question with a question: "Would you write me that prescription for more hours in the day?"

This was my first sign of her humor. I responded, "You can add a good sense of humor to your strengths list."

She flipped the pages back and wrote, "You are funny."

I prompted her to read the second list.

She began reading from the page titled, "What I Would Do If I Had More Hours in the Day or Days in the Week?"

1. Lift weights
2. Walk
3. Eat healthily
4. Lose weight
5. Have my hair done
6. Learn to make myself look pretty
7. Take a singing lesson
8. Redesign my kitchen
9. Write a song
10. Grow an herb garden

I was struck by the contrast of the two lists. "Do you see any differences in your lists?" I asked.

She concluded, "Yes, I obviously am too busy and need more time to have as many items on my strength list as I do on my wish list.

I asked her to look again. "Do you notice a difference in whom your strengths focus on now and whom you would focus on if you had more time?"

Silence.

I continued, "Do you notice that your strengths are in giving to others, and your wish list is devoted to yourself?"

Silence.

"Do you struggle to prioritize time for yourself? Many people do," I offered, "including health professionals, who often find it easier to give to others and believe that caring for themselves is selfish, not as important, or not necessary. What do you think?"

We sat in silence.

Carmen was spinning her fingers on the yellow pad as she slowly spoke. "I guess it's easier caring for others than focusing on me. I am just soft. I don't matter."

Silence.

"My parents," she hesitated, "they called me soft. They said 'soft' with a southern drawl, dragging the word out as if it was a disease. 'You are s-o-f-t,'" she repeated it with a southern accent.

They seemed to know I was different, even before I knew, even before I went to school. My older brother was "strong," and my younger sister was "tough"—both words were given as compliments—but I was "s-o-f-t." They called me Soft Joseph, which when shortened became Sofsef. My father said even my bones were soft. When my brother fell climbing a tree, he bounced back. When I fell from a chair, I broke my arm. Mom said even my skin was soft. When my sister got scratched building a fort, she got a bandage. When I got cut turning a page of my book, I got an infection. Everyone knew I was soft, even the doctor that they forced me to see regularly, even when I felt fine. He seemed to have a "soft" script that I was to follow; he never asked questions but only offered lengthy explanations for my softness. I refused his labels. I rejected the word *soft* and just wanted to be left alone. The name followed me to school, and classmates had contests to see who could make Sofsef cry. I tried hard not to, but in the end I always broke down. My brother despised my being soft and stopped talking to me. My sister worked hard to make me tough, coaching me uselessly to ignore the bullies until she couldn't stand me anymore either.

Tears welled up in Carmen's eyes, and her mascara dripped. She accepted my tissue and covered her face.

She looked up and announced quietly that it was time to go. I thanked her for coming, for committing to her health, and for sharing with me. She thanked me and asked if she could have more questions to answer at home, and if she could come back and talk again. I told her that we would reschedule her physical exam and restated, "It would be my privilege to be your PCP." I ordered her overdue labs and refilled her medications. I gave her two additional lists to create: who and what mattered to her and what she loved. I shared that I would do homework as well and read up on transgender issues. She recommended I read Jennifer Boylan's autobiography, *She's Not There: A Life in Two Genders*.[91] I thanked her and reached to shake her hand. Her circling fingers released her pad of paper and reached back.

After Carmen left my office, I was struck by how difficult it was for her to identify her personal strengths and how hard it was for her to list anything she believed she did well. I ordered the book and did some research to better understand the care needed for patients who are *transgender*—a general term describing people whose gender identity is not fully congruent with their assigned sex at birth. I tried to imagine Carmen's experience growing up and was concerned to see that members of the lesbian, gay, bisexual, transgender, queer, and questioning (LGBTQQ) community have higher rates of all-cause mortality, depression, and suicidal ideation, attempts, and completions compared to the general population.[92-94] Bullying of LGBT youth, often referred to as "gay bashing" or "queer bashing," is a major concern in school systems, where LGBT individuals are three times more likely to be harassed and four times more likely to attempt suicide than other youth.[94] Suicide is already a leading cause of death in fifteen- to twenty-four-year-olds, and causes are linked to bullying, isolation, social stigma, and cultural phobias. A full ninety percent of LGBT students report harassment compared to 62 percent of non-LGBT students, and nearly 40 percent of LGBT youth have attempted suicide at some point. Research is limited, as transgender individuals in the past and present underreport, and death certificates of suicides prior to the 1990s did not consider "sexual orientation" in their data collection or analyses.[95-97]

Over the past decade programs have been initiated to understand and address the needs of LGBT individuals, with a particular aim at reducing suicide among LGBT youth. Interventions are directed toward education, empowerment, acceptance, legal rights, and policy development.[96,98-100] The Family Acceptance Project's research has demonstrated that "parental acceptance or even neutrality, with regard to a child's sexual orientation" can bring down the attempted suicide rate.[101] Schools that include the presence of GSA (gay-straight alliance) programs diminish isolation and have also successfully decreased suicide rates.[102] Reading the limited publications about complex health needs and issues of insurance coverage, I wondered what doctors years ago would have known, asked, or taught patients and what my colleagues now are asking and teaching patients, given the scarcity of training on transgender care in medical school curriculum.[103,104]

When Carmen returned for future visits, we reviewed her medications, weight, blood pressure, blood sugar, and her mood, and each time she proudly presented answers to my questions in the form of lists on her small yellow notepad. Some lists were short, others quite long, but each told a story of who she was. Our discussions were proof of how intensely she considered each question. Each visit was like a window, opening further and further for both of us to clearly see, learn, and care for her.

## Second Visit

On our second visit we talked about her mood, which she reported had recently been down. "Never suicidal," she anticipated my question, "but always low this time of year." She described how she had grown up in Chicago, lived in Wisconsin, and moved to New Hampshire, where the cold, dark winters were all difficult. She wondered why she had never moved to the South, where her family had originated. The top list of her notepad, titled "Who and What Matters to Me," contained only one item.

"Who matters to you?" I inquired.

"My family," she replied.

"Is your family still in Chicago?" I asked.

Silence.

"I don't know," she replied.

With no further prompting, Carmen answered the question I was about to ask: *What was your family's response to your change?* Her words poured out a lifetime of events.

By the time I started school, my parents insisted that there was something medically wrong with me. They repeatedly told the doctor I was gaining weight but not eating, complained of stomach pain, stayed away from social activities, did poorly at school, and was always moody. Tests returned negative, and they concluded my problems were just a "phase" that I would eventually outgrow. In grade school my parents punished me for purchasing a bra and for wasting their money, their time, and my life. My brother made it clear that they were all homophobic, screaming that I was gay and writing "fag" on my door. Even worse was when my sister told her friends that I stole her clothes and dressed like a girl. They were angry and wanted answers. They wanted to define me, to label me, to understand what had gone wrong with me. They wanted someone to blame.

In middle school my family finally agreed that it was okay if I was gay, provided I go for help. I was angry and confused; I refused to go and was unwilling to negotiate their homosexual label. I denied that I was attracted to boys; I denied that I was attracted to girls. I just wanted to be left alone. In high school my mother withdrew from my father. My siblings blamed me for everything that went wrong in the family. They concluded that I was unfixable and agreed that there was nothing they could do to help me. The whole family was on antidepressants, but no one would go to the therapy my doctor recommended. After I graduated from high school, their acceptance came in the form of a truce to ignore me. I moved out at eighteen, relieved to no longer be a burden. Years later I read my sister's engagement announcement in the newspaper and received confirmation in black-and-white print that I no longer existed. The article listed only one brother of the bride-to-be.

Throughout high school, I associated with a small group of computer geeks. They never asked anything of me, and I never offered. A few years after graduation two of them started a computer company and offered me a job. For the next twenty years I was relieved to be living alone, working successfully seven days a week as a computer programmer, and cooking elaborately for myself.

Carmen's family's reaction so closely paralleled the continuum of the stages of grief, described by Elisabeth Kübler-Ross and David Kessler—denial, anger, bargaining, depression, and acceptance—that one could interpret she was dead.[105]

Carmen's words continued to spill.

I searched for answers to my identity confusion, and in my forties read Jennifer Boylan's autobiography. She was the first person I knew who shared my thoughts, and I saw hope for the other me. I was living alone, so there was no one to tell, no one to come out to. I moved to the Upper West Side of Chicago and began dressing as a woman. I felt excitement, contemplated names, and decided on Carmen, which was strong yet feminine. Wearing flowing clothes, I imagined a new me. After attending the dreaded required therapy, I was diagnosed with "gender dysphoria," and I began estrogen treatments that transitioned my body to match my thoughts and emotions.

I began feeling connected and saw opportunities where I might fit in. I tried engaging with co-workers. On one occasion I even RSVP'd yes to a party, but fear of being found out reverted me to past excuses, and I canceled to care for a "sick relative." I gained weight and experienced a curious softening of my muscles and my skin. This felt both female and good and also horrifying, as I fulfilled my parent's prophecy. I was soft.

Carmen sat circling her fingers for what seemed like minutes before she spoke again.

My change in voice was a welcome surprise, and I began to sing in a range not previously possible. I researched transgender options, and at forty-eight began my journey to surgically become transsexual. I moved to Wisconsin, where I met Marla and Cary. They were from Arizona; they were also different, but they were proud to be different and shared their differences openly with everyone. In Wisconsin I shared the same surgeon with Cary and was undergoing similar reassignment. Cary introduced me to Marla, who had completed the surgery and offered her as a resource if I had questions. They spoke openly and eagerly, sometimes in Spanish, which I barely understood. But, being alone, I clung to them both. They became my whole world; everything else was gone. After my surgery I moved in with them and we began calling ourselves "Las Mujeres."

Carmen laughed and ended by saying, "They are my family and they are all that matter." When she looked up, she appeared to have forgotten I was there. She took a deep breath and apologized for the long answer to my question. I thanked her for sharing and, after a pause, asked more about her decision to have surgery, which I had read was rare among those transitioning male to female. Carmen described how they removed "his" testicles and inverted "his" penis to create her vagina and how she was given saline breast implants.

I shared that I had learned: of those transitioning male to female (MTF) only 16–20 percent have had vaginoplasty and breast implants, 20–28 percent prefer not to ever have them, and 54–60 percent report they may have them someday. Of those transitioning female to male (FTM) approximately 40 percent have had breast surgery, 8 percent prefer not to ever, and 51 percent report they may someday. In comparison, only 2 percent report having had phalloplasty (penile implants), 72 percent prefer not to have it, and 26 percent report they may someday. I also inquired about Carmen's sexual orientation, to which she denied ever being sexually active. She was in the minority of 4 percent who identify as asexual. Others were split, with 23 percent reporting they are gay, 24 percent bisexual, 23 percent heterosexual, 23 percent pansexual, and 2 percent other.[106] When I asked what she loved, Carmen responded eagerly, flipping the pages in her notepad and reading from her list titled "Things I Love":

1. Being with Cary and Marla
2. Cooking
3. Singing
4. Teaching colleagues about computers
5. Learning about myself

When she read the list, she was energized. I was thrilled that she found the questions valuable, and I asked her to consider two additional questions. "Take your time," I told her, "as these are fundamental to knowing who you are and your path forward. First, what do you believe is the meaning or purpose of your life? In other words, what unique contribution can you alone make in this world? What would you do for a living if money were not an issue? Second, what are you committed to contributing to and achieving in the future? In other words, what does your vision look like? If you knew you could not fail, what would you like to see happening in five or ten years? How would you like to be remembered?" As I asked the questions, Carmen jotted notes on the top of the next page in her notepad. She left with a dry tissue, and as I reached to shake her hand, she stepped forward and hugged me, as she has done every visit since.

## Third Visit

On her third visit we talked again about her blood pressure, weight, blood sugar, medications, and mood, which she reported had been better recently. She had thought a great deal about her purpose and her future and flipped eagerly to the page titled, "Purpose; The Meaning of My Life." Under the title she had inserted a favorite quote of mine by Henry David Thoreau: "If I am not myself, who else will be?"

Her list was short.

1. To speak and make my voice heard to myself and to others
2. To accept myself, be SOFT, and be me

Without prompting, Carmen began talking about her invisibility. "I used to ask myself, am I a man? But after transitioning I asked myself, am I a woman? A woman in a man's body or a man in a woman's body? I used to think I could hide. When they offered to put me in a box, to be gay, to be soft, or to just disappear, I chose the latter. I became the invisible man," she said. "They operated on my body, but not my mind. I still hid. I looked different to others, but in the mirror my thoughts remained confused. Was I now an invisible woman?"

Carmen sat and stared. I stared back, mindlessly distracted by the young black man in Ralph Ellison's *Invisible Man*.[107] I pictured the character who, fittingly, didn't have a name, spending so many years trying to be who others wanted him to be, only to become invisible not only to others but also to himself. I was struck by her statement and repeated it as a question: "You are the invisible woman?"

"Yes," she offered. "I was packaged in a new body, but it was unknown to me. I was still doing what others thought I should do, which was to 'go away.' I was equally hidden as a woman as I was as a man. Initially, I didn't know the answers to your question of my strengths or what I loved or what mattered to me. It was uncomfortable to consider, but now, as I see a piece of me appearing, I am eager to know who I am and to find my purpose, to use my voice."

She sat silently, her hands circling, her eyes staring down at her list. "I have become hard, not because that is me, but because I was afraid to be soft, afraid to be in their box. I fear I am losing the softness, which was never a disease but a part of me. I'm no longer sure what I want even if I could have it. I have tried to be strong. Men are strong, but I was not a strong man. I tried to be tough. Women are tough, but I am not a tough woman either. What if I actually am soft? Is it okay that I am gentle, kind, accepting? What if I like my softness? What if I have a soft voice and speak it loudly? What if I accept me? Be SOFT, go inside, and be okay with that? What if softness was never a disease? What if it was a part of me that I denied? What if I now want to be me?"

Silence.

"What if?" I echoed, thinking about the game I played with my daughters.

Carmen continued, "I never chose this career. I never loved computers; I went down that path, as it was comfortable. My job is okay, and I make good money, but I dread the thought of doing it forever. When you asked me 'If money weren't an issue, what would I do?' I realized I would quit." She paused and turned the page, showing a long list of items under the title of "Vision: A Future That Could Not Fail":

1. Improve my health
2. Lose weight and lower my blood pressure

3. Eat healthier and lower my blood sugar
4. Improve my mood and get therapy
5. Redesign the kitchen
6. Teach cooking lessons
7. Write a song
8. Sing in a coffee house
9. Change jobs
10. Counsel transgender individuals

"If I knew I could not fail," she continued, "I would take better care of myself. I would do more of the things I love. I would also want to make a difference to others like me. I would coach others to be themselves. I would be a counselor, a transgender counselor. I would be a really strong transgender counselor."

I was so impressed with her insights; her learning was now mine. I congratulated her on not permitting past thoughts to limit her thinking about the future and celebrated the order of her list, which focused first on filling her own tank and then on giving to others. I acknowledged her hard work and encouraged her to use her strengths to achieve her goals. I shared that I believed in her and would be cheering for her as she achieved her vision.

Carmen set out to create a concrete plan and discovered links between past habits of hiding and patterns of poor eating and activity. She made a connection between not feeling cared for and not caring for herself. She made commitments to healthy behaviors and to herself, her mission, and her vision. To this day Carmen continues to take steps forward and to have setbacks. She lost twenty-five pounds the first year and was successful at lowering her blood pressure and eliminating one medication. She lowered her blood sugar, became a much healthier cook, and redesigned her kitchen. During the lengthy construction, she ate out regularly and gained back ten pounds but then refocused on her vision and took the time to write down recipes and to put them into a cookbook. She still struggles to exercise and finds everything except walking to be unpleasant. She is writing songs and has shared many of them with me. She even sings at a local coffee shop, where I hope to someday see her perform. Astoundingly, she also changed her career. She began taking night and online classes, and six months later was interviewing. She now works in social services, counseling at a local nonprofit youth program supporting transgender education for the New England area.

My learning from Carmen continued as I became the physician for all Las Mujeres and was recommended by them to others among our transgender community. Carmen sent me a card thanking me for asking her what matters and for listening to her. "Did you know," the card read, "that 'silent' and 'listen' have the same letters?" Carmen continues on her journey toward personal inquiry, self-awareness, and authenticity. She validated my belief that no matter how much I learn or teach, I continue to gain wisdom by asking questions of myself and others. The committed learner and teacher, who teach and learn together, hold unlimited potential for personal growth and development. She taught me what it really means to be true to oneself and to achieve one's full potential. Carmen thrives in her role as my teacher and has become one of my students' favorite patients, telling and retelling her story over and over again, learning from and teaching all of us.

• • • • • • • • • • • •

HEALTH CHALLENGE #2 | Complete a Self-SWOT

The power to question is the basis for all human progress.
GANDHI

Develop the habit of lifelong learning and discover who you are. Apply the Socratic method of inquiry to increase self-awareness and promote personal wellness. Devote fifteen minutes a day for the next thirty days to consider fundamental questions, complete a self-SWOT, and create a personal mission and vision statement. Review the following questions and revise your answers continuously to understand and direct aspects of your life and your health. Create lists, as Carmen did, or write short descriptive essays, depending on your strengths, skills, and preference. Questions can also be used to increase awareness of another person.

SELF-SWOT    The SWOT assessment tool is invaluable in reflecting on strengths, weaknesses, opportunities, and threats (SWOT). Complete a self-SWOT after finishing a project, a major life milestone, a challenging day, or at the end of every year. Continually revisit your SWOTs and analyze them

| My strengths | My weaknesses |
|---|---|
| My opportunities | My threats |

Adapted from SWOT analysis template—a free resource from
www.businessballs.com. Template © Alan Chapman 2004.

to renew and change goals for improvement. The SWOT worksheet below can be used to record your responses and will be revisited in future lessons.

1. Strengths: What do you think you do well? What do others say you do well? Consider your unique knowledge, skills, beliefs, and style. Consider your fortes in balancing your own health and caring for others.
2. Weaknesses: What do you believe are your gaps? What do others say you could do better? Consider areas where you fall short in authenticity, integrity, commitments, or performance.
3. Opportunities: What would you do if you had more hours in the day and days in the week? Consider resources and activities that you might take advantage of to promote your strengths. What weaknesses could you consider as potential goals for self-improvement?
4. Threats: What limits your effectiveness? What intrinsic and extrinsic factors prohibit your strengths or accentuate your weaknesses?

MISSION AND VISION STATEMENT   These statements, like the SWOT, can be applied to individuals or organizations and are invaluable in discovering who you are and contributing to your fullest potential. They can also be used on a daily basis to drive your efforts and maintain focus on what matters. Create your personal statements by answering the following questions:

1. Mission: What are you passionate about? What do you love that brings you joy and peace? Consider how this affects your health. What is your purpose? What do you believe is the meaning of your life? What unique contribution can you alone make in this world? What would you do for a living if money were not an issue?
2. Vision: What are your future priorities? Who and what matter most to you? If all else went away, what would be critical to your world? Take into account the influence of these priorities on your health and well-being. What are you committed to contributing to? What would you like to see yourself doing or achieving in one, three, five, and ten years if you knew you could not fail? How would you like to be feeling and what healthy lifestyle would you be living?

• ◆ ● • • • • • • • ◆ ●

# BUILD RESILIENCE

*The human spirit is stronger than anything that can happen to it.*
GEORGE C. SCOTT

I have been caring for Nelle since I began practicing, over twenty years ago. When she joined my panel of patients, she had only one diagnosis, somewhat unusual for a patient in her midseventies. Nelle is a petite, feisty lady; a zesty, spirited, and irrepressible woman, who has lived a life full of challenges and opportunities. I admire how Nelle has embraced hardships in life as if they were her friends. Nothing can shake her; nothing can dampen her day; nothing can break her spirit. Her smile surrounds her like a protective shield. Negative experiences seemed to slide off her, as if she were coated in Teflon. Even in her nineties, Nelle's energy, positivity, and outlook on life inspire and bring energy to those around her.

Nelle described her childhood adversity matter-of-factly, reframing the negative by focusing on the positive. It seemed almost unreal that, given her upbringing, she harbored no anger, no resentment, and no negative thoughts. When she spoke of the strength she acquired after her father's suicide, I asked her how she viewed loss so positively and what, if anything, in her life she perceived as difficult.

Nelle shared with me that, days before her fiftieth birthday, she had faced her greatest struggle. She was driving her first husband to receive chemotherapy for his colon cancer, ran a red light, and hit a parked car. In the ambulance to the hospital, she recalled a sharp pain in her right eye, and at that moment the world went dark. She feared her husband wouldn't get his treatment. The emergency-room doctor diagnosed her with optic neuritis and asked extensive questions about past neurologic symptoms. "Have you experienced any numbness, weakness, tingling, falls?" he probed. She recalled two previous episodes: the first was a weakness in her right arm and the second was a feeling of electric shock running down her neck; both of them lasted a few days but then resolved. On the basis of her symptoms, the doctor suspected multiple sclerosis (MS). He referred her to a neurologist, who ordered an MRI scan, and confirmed the diagnosis.

Nelle read everything available on MS and felt fortunate to learn that she had "relapsing remitting" MS, the most common and most benign type. She shared how she felt fortunate to begin treatment quickly and to return to her activities in weeks compared to the months of prolonged chemotherapy and radiation that her husband received. She was advised that interferon immunotherapy would help prevent the progression of her fatigue and was grateful to find how fast steroids worked to recoup her energy. When her husband died, she vowed to stay as healthy as possible in his honor.

Over the years stresses provoked exacerbations, just as she had been told to expect, but Nelle would not be broken. She said, "MS is my built-in reminder to take special care of myself," acknowledging she had previously been focusing on her husband's health rather than on her own. She immediately began walking daily, which for years she had been doing only intermittently, and she declared that she had a "chronic disease," not a "terminal one." She continued to see a neurologist once a year, viewing that visit as her "tune up." To Nelle MS became an opportunity to listen to her body. When she was fatigued, she napped. When she was in pain, she permitted herself a day off. When she had weakness in her right arm, she focused on walking or healthy eating. When she had visual changes, she would listen to audiobooks and later celebrate the boost of energy that followed a course of steroids. She seemed to accept anything and everything that came her way. In my office one day, she told me how having MS allowed her to connect with all her aging friends whose lives centered on their multitudes of health conditions. "Without MS," she said, "I would not fit in."

## What Is Resilience?

Nelle never described herself as resilient, but she is perhaps the most resilient person I have ever encountered. Experts have studied the concept of resilience for decades. The American Psychological Association defines resilience as "the process of adapting well in the face of adversity, trauma, threats, and even significant sources of stress—such as family and relationship problems, serious health problems or workplace and financial stresses."[108] Resilience is thought to be critical to one's success in navigating all aspects of life. In a 2002 *Harvard Business Review* article, Diane Coutu summarizes her extensive research around resilience with a quote from a CEO she interviewed: "More than education, more than experience, more than training, a person's resilience will determine who succeeds and who fails. That's true in the cancer wards, it's true in the Olympics, it's true in the boardroom."[109]

Resiliency is a critical topic in health care today for three reasons. First, knowledge is expanding. The fields of neuroscience, physiology, psychology, and genetics are advancing the understanding of trauma and stress and the impact of resilience in preventing and addressing short- and long-term health consequences. Second, rising levels of chronic stress, anxiety, depression, and the current epidemic of burnout demand we address solutions. Third, and most important, while no blood test or gene for resilience exists to date, experts collectively believe that evidence-based strategies for building resilience can be taught and learned. In other words, the potential to build resilience exists, and it can be demonstrated within each one of us. The challenge is to tap into it and to do so prior to needing it.

The landmark Adverse Childhood Experiences Study looked broadly at the determinants of health and concluded that children exposed to bad situations early in life were destined to high-risk behaviors and poor health outcomes.[20] Vincent Felitti and his colleagues investigated children with histories of abuse and family dysfunction and found they were at extremely high risk for negative outcomes the rest of their lives. They established a strong correlation between adverse childhood experiences and the subsequent development, during the teenage years, of high-risk behaviors, legal problems, poor health outcomes, and physical and mental disorders. Teens with adverse childhood experiences went on to have higher incidences of chronic health conditions and ultimately higher morbidity and mortality as adults by comparison to those without such adversity.

Norman Garmezy, a child psychologist at the University of Minnesota, was one of the earliest researchers to use the term *resilient*. Garmezy and other researchers studied children who defied Felitti's observed patterns of poor outcomes. They observed exceptional children who excelled beyond expectations despite horrific experiences, to identify protective factors that contributed to their resilience.[110] In 1989 Emmy Werner completed a thirty-year study of middle school students tagged as "at risk" and found that while, as Felitti predicted, nearly two-thirds went on to demonstrate high-risk behaviors, a minority defied expectations and succeeded beyond anyone's beliefs. The resilient one-third attained academic, domestic, and social success and developed into "competent, confident, and caring young adults."[111]

Many factors contribute to one's ability to not only survive but thrive in the face of adversity, and every day we hear examples of unbreakable individuals. Jaycee Dugard, in her memoir, *Freedom: My Book of Firsts*, remains "positive" and "purposeful" beyond comprehension after being kidnapped at age eleven and held in captivity until her emancipation eighteen years later. She focused on "finding meaning" in her liberated life. She began the JAYC Foundation to support families who have suffered trauma and says, "Some terrible thing happened to me, but I am not going to let it ruin the rest of my life."[112] In a 2016 article the journalist Susie Neilson described her interview with Johnny Perez, a prisoner who spent thirteen years in prison and three years of his sentence in solitary confinement. Perez was "resourceful," unlike other prisoners who have gone "insane" in isolation, and reported that "he left a better man." He described committing his time to "creating imagery, completing mental and physical exercises, journaling his story, and meditating to tap into and develop a stronger sense of self."[113]

Post-traumatic stress disorder (PTSD) is a syndrome of reactions experienced by many after trauma. *Resilience*, among other terms, has been described as the power to avoid PTSD. In contrast, PTG, or post-traumatic growth, is one's ability to benefit from an adverse experience. The designation *potentially traumatic event* (PTE), coined by clinical psychologist George Bonanno, head of the Loss, Trauma, and Emotion Lab at Columbia University, critically distinguishes individuals' capacity to thrive post adversity based on their "perception of the event." [114] In other words, the way in which one views the traumatic experiences determines the degree to which one is negatively or positively affected—the degree to which one is resilient.

## How Do We Build Resilience?

A compelling summary of research on resilience factors is *Resilience: The Science of Mastering Life's Greatest Challenges*, by Drs. Steven M. Southwick and Dennis S. Charney.[7] These psychiatrists from Yale University interviewed Vietnam POWs, U.S. Army Special Force instructors, and a diverse group of civilians who had experienced a broad range of intense stresses. The authors integrated psychological and neuroscience research with stories about those who succeeded against all odds. They identified ten factors, practiced in no particular order, believed to be attainable by all. I have had the privilege of co-teaching resiliency training to medical colleagues with Dr. Southwick, highlighting each factor as a strategy that can be applied to build resilience. Being a doctor requires resilience: the more resilient, the better the doctor. This is true perhaps now more than ever, as conflicting demands have led to high levels of stress.

While Drs. Southwick and Charney's work focused on individuals, their strategies can and must be adapted to build resilience across teams, organizations, and communities. It is now widely recognized across the medical field that resilience training across all ages and disciplines fosters protection and motivation to engage in challenges at work.[115,116] But only when these strategies are successfully applied broadly to overcome the chronic stress and burnout in health professionals will we be able to maximize care for patients. Individuals and leaders in the health-care system have a responsibility to implement programs and provide resources to grow resilience within our curriculums and across our practices. In the 2013 *Academic Medicine* article "Physician Resilience: What It Means, Why It Matters, and How to Promote It," resilience experts Drs. Ronald Epstein and Michael Krasner summarize recent research and make a call for action: "It is in the self-interest of health care institutions to support the efforts of all members of the health care workforce to enhance their capacity for resilience; it will increase quality of care while reducing errors, burnout, and attrition."[115,116]

I give Dr. Southwick's book as a gift to students, colleagues, family, and friends and recommend it to all, as no one is immune to life's stresses. I shared it with Nelle, briefly reviewing the ten factors, and asked her, as I do with other patients, to assess her own resilience. I asked her to place the ten items on a self-SWOT worksheet and to rate each of the factors in relation to her on a scale of 1 to 5, with 1 being "not at all," and 5 being "extremely." "The goal," I explained, "is to understand your strengths, weaknesses, opportunities, and threats and then to prioritize areas for personal improvement." Nelle scored herself a 47 out of the possible 50 and was perhaps the only one I know who placed all ten factors under "strengths."

I assess my own resilience using these ten factors and the SWOT tool (see lesson 2) regularly, and while my strength box is by no means as full as Nelle's, I continually find new ways to minimize my weaknesses and threats and convert my opportunities into strengths. I see how the presence or absence of factors affects my health and the health of others. In assessing my own resilience, I remind myself that I don't need to be strong in all areas to be resilient. Most of the time my natural strengths serve me well. But under time constraints and increased stress, I can find ways to double-dip, for instance, running with colleagues to build my physical health and social supports.

At age eighty Nelle had outlived two husbands; the first died of colon cancer, the second of heart disease. She, on the other hand, was thriving: She lived alone, maintained a small motor home, and functioned totally independently. She served meals at the senior center and laughed as she shared that she was older than most of the patrons. She stayed physically and mentally active by walking, doing Sudoku, and sewing crafts for local summer markets and holiday bazaars. I am the proud recipient of many of her creations, which are innovative and quite functional, like my beautifully sewn "bag sleeve" that dispenses plastic grocery bags and my "bracelet gadget" that clasps a bracelet on one hand by linking the two ends together, a task otherwise nearly impossible. She also creates male and female dolls, paints note cards boasting famous sayings and off-color jokes, and crochets holiday ornaments. I share her jokes with staff, and they are shocked that they come from an octogenarian.

At eighty-three Nelle remained a healthy widow and established a new relationship with a "male friend" named Simon. She knew him for years as an energetic and engaged member of the senior-center community, but only two years later she again found herself a caregiver. I wondered if Nelle's role as a caregiver also contributed to her resilience or if her resilience made her a natural caregiver. Simon's mild dementia progressed and required his transition to a nursing home. Nelle visited him daily, telling him stories to keep his spirit alive. She admitted that many days he didn't recognize her, but she believed that her presence made a difference for him and joked that her time with him also "kept her out of trouble." When Nelle was eighty-seven, Simon passed away.

At ninety Nelle's eyesight continued to diminish. I feared this would be a breaking point. She could no longer thread her needles and would have to relinquish her driver's license and with it her independence. Not a chance. She befriended a young neighbor whom she described as "techy, lonely, and dependable." She took on the role of mentor, and she allowed herself to be mentored. She was introduced to Facebook, purchased an iPad, and got "connected." She began receiving photos from her children and grandchildren. While she never mastered sending pictures, she felt enormous joy in seeing photos from her family. Nelle also recruited admirers like myself who supplied her with prethreaded sewing kits acquired from hotels.

At ninety-one Nelle was my oldest patient and one of the few for whom I had cared since I began practice. That year Nelle developed pneumonia, as many elderly patients do. When I was a medical student, my senior physicians often told me pneumonia was "the old man's best friend." These mentors shared that when elderly patients get pneumonia, "they go peacefully, they go comfortably, and they go quickly." I was *not* ready for Nelle to go at all and strongly recommended she be admitted to the hospital, where she could be monitored and cared for. Nelle declined. She declared that she was not afraid to go when it was her time. She said I should keep the hospital bed open in case a "young'un" might need it and that she was sure we had better uses for our fancy medical technology than taking care of her. She was alert, competent, and had clear directives to avoid heroic measures. Besides, she told me, she was excited that her granddaughter Helen from Ohio would be coming to visit for the next two weeks.

Nelle's pneumonia was a reminder to me of how quickly life changes, how precious life is, and how things we value can disappear in an instant. My own grandmother passed away in her sleep when I was in medical school. As Nelle left my office that afternoon, I feared I wouldn't see her again. I sat in my office that evening dictating a detailed medical note. After documenting her respiratory rate, oxygen-saturation level, informed consent, and level of competency, I continued to write. I wrote what I felt, what I had learned from Nelle, what she had generously shared in pieces over the years. I wrote from my heart, not for the chart. I wrote a poem about Nelle. Later that week I made a house call, a practice that is still justified for patients who are elderly and homebound. I wanted to bring Nelle a gift, something valuable to a ninety-one-year-old who has everything. I gave her my poem.

## I Admire You

BY CATHERINE F. PIPAS, MD

I admire you,
Every time I see you, you are a teacher to me, a role model
You who are my patient
You who have grown with me for the past twenty years
You who own ninety-one years of experience
You with your holiday color–coordinated clothing
You who still care for the elderly and cook for seniors
You who sew crafts through magnifying glasses for holiday fund-raisers
You who handwrite jokes of every color and style to share with me at
    every visit
You who have only one medical problem
You who find no fault in the world
You with your positive attitude
You whom I hope to emulate as I age

I admire you,
As I have gotten to know you and learned your story
You who were adopted
You who no one wanted as a baby
You who landed in a home of three adopted children
You who were burned in order to potty train
You who were never the favored child
You who were sexually abused by your "mother's" father
You who felt expected to do it all
You who separated the fighting sisters but never cried
You who cleaned up the remains of your "father's" suicide
You who cared for your aging mother

I admire you,
For all that life has given you, and all you have given to life
You, who still eat your breakfast, like a "good girl"
You who tell yourself "I'll show them"
You who observe but do not judge
You who laugh at all the world
You who didn't just survive, but thrived
You who speak your mind and feel your feelings
You whose generosity has no limits
You who focus on the half-full portion of the glass
You who are committed to goodness
You whose story will be told over and over by me

Nelle beamed with pride as I read it aloud. She asked me to read it again for Helen, who joined us and held Nelle's hand and cried. Nelle, as it turned out, was not the "old man" in need of a best friend, nor was she, as she claimed, an "old woman." In the end, pneumonia would not break her but would be one more challenge that she turned into an opportunity. Nelle rested, enjoyed Helen's company, and recovered fully. On her follow-up office visit, she updated me on her granddaughter's trip back to Ohio and her own return to cooking at the senior center. She reported she was feeling better now than she had in years. Nelle was nearing her ninety-second birthday and I my fiftieth when she sat in my office that day. I was relieved by her energy but remained apprehensive, thinking that any visit could be our last. I was mindful of Nelle's resilience and hoped that the richness of her accumulated wisdom and generosity would stay with me forever.

Last month, at ninety-three years old and one year after her bout of pneumonia, Nelle was back for a visit. She shared that she had sent my poem to her three children. Each subsequently wrote me notes, expressing their appreciation of my caring for and honoring their mother. Her eldest son wrote, "Thank you for your wonderful tribute to my mom. She is wonderful and loving. I cherish her every day. She has been through a lot, and I have shared many of the good and bad times with her. I admire you for writing this about my mom. Thank you, Jason." To this day Nelle is alive and well. I am still trying to bottle the "essence of Nelle." I continue my search to capture her secret, to know her better, to benefit personally, and to reproduce her spirit for others.

We are all exposed at some point in our lives to personal loss, physical or emotional health complications, complex social situations, harsh environments, financial difficulties, or issues of inequality. The challenge is to build resilience across our lifetime so that we, like Nelle, have the capability to optimize well-being by transforming our challenges into opportunities and preparing for future adversity.

• • • • • • • • • • • •

HEALTH CHALLENGE #3    Perform a Self-Assessment

*Our greatest glory is not in never falling, but in getting up every time we do.*
CONFUCIUS

Revisit your self-SWOT from lesson 2 and assess yourself on each of Dr. Southwick's following ten factors by placing each factor within one of the four quadrants. For example, if you are positive in your thinking, then "optimism" will go in your strengths quadrant. If you tend toward negative thinking, "optimism" may be a threat to your success, or if you are motivated to improve it through appreciative inquiry, it may be an opportunity. How many of the ten are your strengths? As you place these factors in your SWOT, place a number next to each to indicate the degree to which you currently possess the factor and a second number to indicate the degree to which the factor is important to you now. Use the following scale for both questions on all ten factors.

1 = not at all; 2 = somewhat; 3 = moderately; 4 = very; 5 = extremely

For example, on factor number 7, physical exercise, you may record a 1 to indicate you exercise "not at all," followed by a 5 to indicate physical activity is "extremely" important to you.

1. Optimism: To what degree do you see the positive in people, problems, or situations? (The Life Orientation Test is a formal ten-item measure of optimism.)

2. Facing fear: To what degree are you committed to understanding, discussing, and addressing that which is stressful and overwhelming to you?

3. Moral compass: To what degree do you display self-discipline and do the right thing even when nobody's watching and even if there are negative consequences?

4. Religion and spirituality: To what degree do you believe in a higher spiritual power and rely on prayer, meditation, or mindfulness to overcome what may seem hopeless?

5. Social support: To what degree do you capitalize on a network of family and friends for support?

6. Role models: To what degree do you have of at least one continuous mentor from whom you gain personal strength, guidance, and insight?

7. Physical exercise: To what degree do you engage in regular exercise?

8. Mental exercise: To what degree do you regularly stimulate your mind by reading, problem solving, or participating in other mental activities?

9. Flexibility and acceptance: To what degree are you able to learn from mistakes, accept what is not perfect, and willingly adapt different styles and strategies to different situations?

10. Meaning and purpose: To what degree are you clear about and willing to defend and not compromise on that which you stand for?

• ● ● ▸ ● ● ● ● ● ● ●

# WRITE YOUR STORY

Knowing yourself is the beginning of all wisdom.
ARISTOTLE

## August 2014

"Excuse me, Dr. Pipas." Sarah interrupted me while I was writing notes. "Ms. Douglas is twenty minutes late for her appointment?" Sarah is completing her first year as a medical student and has been shadowing me every Tuesday afternoon for the past twelve months. Her presence is a reminder to my patients and me of our roles as teachers, and she has become the ears, eyes, and heart of my office.

Sarah's voice was unusually hesitant when she interrupted. Her statement, disguised as a question, exposed her fear. "I tried her home but got no answer." Sarah remained at the door, her dark-brown eyes searching mine for reassurance. She had seen Lee monthly with me over the past year and knew her nearly as well as I did. Lee is never late. My mind raced to her past visits. Remember! Remember! I plead with myself. What was her plan? What choice had she made? Sarah redialed her home phone, and I pulled up Lee's medical record on the computer. I reviewed her chart as my mind jumped to her visit a year ago.

## August 2013

Lee's visit on that scorching hot day the previous summer began like all visits but ended miles from where I had anticipated. At that time I had been her primary-care doctor for four years. She presented for follow-up hypertension and was the first patient Sarah and I saw that Tuesday afternoon. Lee is a gentle woman in her late sixties with snow-white hair, china-doll skin, and delicate features. Her smile is contagious, her hugs warm, and her hands soft. She was dressed in an elegant two-piece tan linen pantsuit, crisply pressed, with matching shoes and a lavender silk scarf that gently wrapped around her graceful neck. She wore a simple chain with a small silver bear, which she said symbolized "courage and strength." Lee claimed "Mother Earth" as her religion, having grown up in Tucson alongside Native Americans. Lee, a psychologist, now retired from practice as a mental-health counselor, lived with her husband, Martin. She stayed active mentally, and that day she carried a copy of *Wild Swans*, a story of three generations of strong Chinese women, which she insisted on passing on to me and which remains one of my favorites.[117]

Lee arrived at appointments promptly and took her medication like clockwork. That day, as on every visit, she proudly presented her meticulously recorded blood-pressure log. As usual, her body weight was ideal and her healthy eating, nonsmoking habits, and daily trips to the gym were unchanged. With her blood pressure well controlled and her preventive care up to date, we had time to discuss her favorite subject: Frances, her adopted daughter, who lived in Arizona with Lee's two grandchildren, Michael and Molly. On that visit Lee shared photos of Molly's recent wedding. Lee had flown there two weeks before to share in the preparations. Lee dreamed about moving back to that beautiful land to be among her family. Then, suddenly, in my office on that hot afternoon, Lee's snow-white skin went ashen like a corpse's, and she began sobbing.

"What happened?" I interrupted her sobs.

"A perfect wedding," Lee said.

I reached for Lee's hand and watched her tears flow, imagining her joy. But Lee's tears were not happy tears; she grasped my hand and slumped in her chair. Her tears shifted to a whimper, a muffled sound, and then to words: "I should never have come back. . . . I can't please him. . . . Martin is never happy. . . . He blames me for everything."

In my surprise I could only reflect Lee's words back to her. "You should never have come back?"

Silence.

Lee sat, her eyes glazed over, as if she had returned to Arizona. Her body slumped, her words were barely audible, and her sobs flowed.

"He hates Arizona, he hates Frances, and he hates me. I should never have come back!" Her words and tears poured out. "His plane was delayed. He missed the wedding. He came into the reception screaming. He said it was my fault: that I booked the flights too close. He's done this so many times, but never to my family, never to my Molly. He yells all the time and expects me to fix everything. I try so hard to do what he wants, always, everything he wants, but this time I wasn't focused on him. I should have checked his flight—it was my fault, I should have taken care of him. I just wanted to be with my family, my Molly." Her words continued to pour out. "No one visits me. I can't go anywhere. He joined my church group. He hates church. He reads my emails, checks my cell phone, and he sold my car. You are the only person I can talk to without him."

I was stunned. I thought I knew Lee, but I had missed knowing Lee's story. The Lee I had previously known was gone. A new Lee was here, living a life that I recognized all too well. My mind flashed to Harriet, a woman I cared for many years ago, a thirty-five-year-old mother of three children. "Trauma," read the death certificate. She and her five-year-old son were found at home with contusions and fractures. Abuse had never been documented in her chart. She had never mentioned a word to me. I later learned that she had gone back to her husband to protect her children, perhaps believing that as long as she was the recipient of his anger, they would be spared. I still grieve for her. My thoughts returned to Lee. This time I would make a difference. I glanced at Sarah and reflexively began drilling Lee. "Are you safe? Has he hurt you? Hit you?" My words were like a splash in her face. Her faraway gaze passed. She stood up and apologized.

"I'm sorry. I'm so sorry for using so much of your time. Never mind." Lee closed up, like an oyster shell, sealing before me as I reached out to touch it. "No, no, no, he is a good man. He loves me. We have a strong marriage. I have to go home and cook. Never mind." She adjusted her perfectly straight silk scarf. "He never hits me. I am safe: I have a good home, a good man."

I was stunned at how quickly her story of trauma had unfolded and how equally swiftly it was wrapped up. "A good man?" I reflected uncomfortably, feeling her ambivalence. Her twenty-minute appointment was over, but more was needed. Today Sarah would learn that an appointment slot could never dictate human need. My waiting patients knew that I would also give them the time they needed. "Tell me more about Martin," I asked. "When did you first meet him?"

But that visit one year ago ended with Lee nodding and repeating, "I am safe. I really am safe." She had agreed to a follow-up in one week but was noncommittal about contacting any of the resources we offered, such as the National Domestic Violence Hotline, and she refused written materials.[118] Lee agreed to be called at home, provided that Sarah and I said we were calling only to check her blood pressure. Lee also agreed that if we arranged for our local domestic violence experts (WISE) to come to my office during her next visit, she would talk with them. Lee left the office but remained on my mind until I saw her the following week.

## August 2014

Sarah interrupted my thoughts of that visit a year ago to let me know the next patient was ready. "Still no word from Lee," she reported. Together we saw the next patient, but my mind returned to Lee. Had Sarah tried all Lee's phone numbers? Should I wait? Call the police? Her daughter? Where was she? We finished with our last patient and our notes but still had heard no word from Lee. As we were leaving for the evening, there was a message flashing on the phone. It was from Martin. He said, "I am returning Dr. Pipas's call regarding Lee Douglas. Lee has gone to Arizona but should be back shortly; she must have forgotten about the appointment." He would give her the message. Sarah's expression mirrored my thoughts. *Is he lying? Is she hurt?* I searched Lee's chart and found a number for her daughter, Frances. No answer. I left a message and asked Lee to call me. "Nothing urgent," I said. "Just a follow-up from her office visit." But as I hung up, I thought to myself that it would be urgent if Lee was not with her. As we walked out, Sarah asked me why I thought abuse happened to so many people. She asked, "Doesn't Lee see the patterns? Isn't she a therapist herself?"

Sarah had read my thoughts. "Yes," I told Sarah. "Lee is an expert, but having knowledge doesn't guarantee we are self-aware or can easily change. I know many physicians who struggle to apply what they know to themselves, including an oncologist who still smokes."

## September 2013

On her follow-up visit a week later, Martin insisted on accompanying Lee to her appointment and sat in the waiting area. Lee was visibly agitated, shifting in her chair, and glancing at her watch. "I mustn't keep him waiting," she said. "Mustn't upset him." She insisted on skipping the physical exam and the prearranged meeting with WISE. She apologized and promised to come alone next time. She shared that after her last visit, Martin had pressured her to stop being so needy. When she told him that talking to her doctor was helpful, he was infuriated and smashed another of her mother's teacups. He told her it was her mom's fault that she needed so much help. He demanded she break ties with that "dead woman" and insisted he was all she needed. Lee stayed in her room for three days, crying and fearing she was becoming her mother. She described how Martin came to her door every hour, apologizing and offering to go to counseling again. He defended himself, saying that he loved her and he would protect her from the memories seeded in her mother's teacups.

Lee slid back into her chair, and the tears again flowed. "I can't do this anymore. I am failing again. We have seen therapists, and all he does is blame everything on me. It is just like my last marriage. I am failing again. We should divorce, but nothing will be different. I am the problem. Why am I like this?" Her words ended, but her tears continued to flow. She regained her composure and shared that she knew the relationship was unhealthy, as her parents' and her first marriage had been. She asked, "Why do I care more about him than myself? Why am I the way I am?"

I held Lee's trembling hand. "Lee, you are a survivor! You have developed coping skills to fit your experiences. These behaviors have kept you alive. In abusive situations survivors' reactions are often extreme: denying basic needs, isolating oneself from others, and, paradoxically, caring for the abuser. These coping skills that kept you alive, unfortunately, can also leave you vulnerable."

"Has either of you read Dr. Judith Herman's book *Trauma and Recovery*?" I asked both Lee and Sarah.[119]

Lee nodded and Sarah shook her head from side to side.

"Do you keep a journal?" I asked them both.

Both shook their heads.

Having been a mental-health counselor, Lee knew where I was headed. She knew that healing and recovery from trauma often included reconstruction of the adverse events through oral or written narratives. She was familiar with Dr. Herman's work, helping survivors explore their pasts, understand the impact of events, validate their own responses, and restore their self-worth. Lee also knew Jamie Pennebaker's book, *Opening Up: The Healing Power of Expressing Emotions*, which correlates the process of post-trauma writing with long-term health.[120]

"Are you willing to reread these, looking at your experiences?" I asked Lee. Lee nodded.

"Are you willing to journal your story?"

She nodded again.

Writing a personal narrative takes courage and must be a conscious decision. It can be a powerful way to restore your sense of personal value and purpose. I shared how writing in my journal is a gift I give myself, how my journal is not to be graded or critiqued by anyone, including me; it is the home of my story, a place where I make sense of my experiences and discover why I am who I am.

"When you are ready," I suggested to Lee, "look at the process in steps. Start by identifying critical experiences in your life. They can be good or bad. Next, reconstruct each event, trying to separate the facts from how you may have interpreted them. For example, a fact may be 'My parents divorced.' My interpretation could be 'It was my fault.' Last, examine thoughts that recur for you after this event, and any feelings or actions that you demonstrate as a result of your thinking. For example, after saying to yourself, 'I can't do anything right' or 'My family is ruined,' you may feel isolated or lonely, or become disengaged.

Lee nodded with each step. "I'm ready. I need to do this, and know my feelings and thoughts are all tangled." She sighed and agreed to follow up in one month, then left for the waiting room, where Martin sat impatiently waiting.

October 2013

Lee surprised both Sarah and me when she returned a month later with a beautiful leather journal, offering to share her story. "I reread Dr. Herman's book and have been writing nonstop," she declared. "I saw my own abusive relationships for the first time and, as you suggested, how my interpretation of those experiences has shaped who I am.

"What did you learn?" I asked.

Lee smiled and read her story:

Father died in his eighties of a heart attack and Mom at seventy-nine of a stroke. I didn't go back to Arizona for either of the funerals. Maybe I should have? Father was a businessman and traded with Native Americans across the Southwest. Mom called herself a homemaker, but Father said she never learned to make a home. He criticized her dry meals, underpressed shirts, and unorganized closets. When he wasn't traveling, Father drank and stomped around, complaining and slamming doors. Everyone walked on eggshells, but I could anticipate his storms and would steam dry chicken, press his shirts, and organize the house. His nickname for me was "Sunny." He boasted that I never caused trouble and was the one he could depend on. My reward was to accompany him on business trips. I loved to go and listen as the Natives told stories, gave him gifts, and then, as he put it, "finally got around to making deals." I loved how the wise elder women shared their stories. I vowed to read and tell stories like them. I vowed to never be like Mom, who couldn't read.

On three occasions police came to our house. The neighbors reported screams, but by the time I returned home from school, Father and the police chief (the brother of one of Father's partners) were in the front yard chatting about land deals. I knew if I had been home before him, I could have kept Mom safe. She locked herself in her room every morning and most evenings. The only memory I have of her smiling is at afternoon tea, a tradition that started after I began kindergarten. We wrapped her silk scarfs around our shoulders and held our pinkies up, imitating British royalty. I still have Mom's teacups.

Lee looked up from her journal and reflected aloud: "Everyone viewed me as dependable. Father needed to be taken care of, and Mom was incapable. I see how I interpreted Father as strong and Mom as weak. I see how I took on her role to protect her. I believed my marriage was different, but I see now how similar Martin is to Father and I to Mom." Lee continued to read:

> I applied to college. Father was aloof, and Mom repeatedly suggested I attend the University of Arizona–Tucson. Worried that Mom needed me, I stayed in Tucson. That time was memorable only for a brief marriage, a briefer divorce, and the fact that I never graduated college. That marriage was a "bad fit" and prompted me to leave Arizona. I began again as a student in Vermont. I was alone until two months later, when I met Martin.
>
> Martin was a security guard and older than me by eight years. He was handsome, gentlemanly, and represented the law. He brought me daisies and poems in the library after his shift. He waited for me to finish studying and escorted me home. He loved to hike, read, and travel, and, most important, he loved children. I was eager to have my own family, and we married a year later. Seven months after the wedding, Martin was nearly killed in a car accident. That was when I realized he drank. His police buddies appeared at the accident, and no DWI was recorded. He was more like my father and my first husband than I cared to recall. After five years of trying to get pregnant, I learned that Martin never liked hiking, reading, or traveling, and he had never wanted children. Martin drunkenly confessed that he had been married previously and had gotten a vasectomy. He begged forgiveness and offered to go with me to counseling. We had two sessions, and he offered to adopt. I wanted to believe he was truly sorry and was thrilled to have baby Frances.

Again Lee looked up from her journal. I prodded her to continue.

> I worked hard to please Martin, perhaps out of fear or a desire to be better than my mom. I was convinced that I could work harder than Mom had done and save my marriage. I see now how my views were

twisted, and how we both focused on our spouse. I now see how I interpreted others' inability to care for me as cause for me to care for them. I brought this misconception into my marriage. I never spoke to anyone about this, not even my brother, who had his own misinterpretations.

Lee looked up briefly and continued to read:

My older brother, Brad, told me that Father treated Mom the way Mom deserved. He repeated Father's role himself. Brad was angry and uncontrollable. He escaped from home at eighteen, went to college, and never came back. Even on holidays he had an excuse for not showing up. At thirty-two he was convicted of beating his girlfriend and her two-year-old son. Perhaps I knew this would happen and feared the same from Martin. I wanted to stay safe myself and keep Martin out of trouble.

Lee ended her story with tears in her eyes. I hugged her and thanked her for sharing. Her voice wavered as she spoke again: "It was hard to write my story and hard to share it, but I wish I had done it earlier. Counseling others, in comparison, was easy. I wish I'd have known more about myself. A friend in college once told me I was crazy for tolerating Martin. She said my 'sweetness' was as uncomfortable for her as his 'bullying.' She told me she would have left Martin on day one, but that she saw how he fit me like a glove. I never responded to her and our friendship ended."

Lee's story paralleled the cycle of power and control and highlighted for me the importance of reflecting on personal narrative to increase self-awareness and achieve personal wellness. When we identify (or someone else points out) unhealthy patterns of behavior, self-reflection is key to deeper understanding. Gaining new knowledge and skills is necessary but not sufficient. Thinking critically about our experiences and how we interpret them provides insight into what drives our feelings, thoughts, and actions. Writing a personal narrative is a powerful and purposeful strategy for knowing *why* we are who we are and exploring our past, present, and future.

I discussed with Lee and Sarah the cycle of control and power, which begins when abusers impose power, fear, or control over victims, who innately try to avoid the abuse but are often not successful without appeasing abusers and giving back control. Thus, a cycle evolves. Abusers frequently show remorse for aggressive behaviors and shower victims with apologies, rewards, or gifts. Victims subsequently feel special and develop a sense of hope or renewed desire to sustain the relationship. Victims make an even greater commitment to protecting or caring for abusers, interpreting them either as needy or as heroes to emulate. The cycle continues, and abusers protect their power by isolating victims and threatening to dissolve past and present contacts through fear or embarrassment. This results in a greater dependency of victims on abusers. Victims, now alone with a secret, are further distanced from other trusting relationships. The last part of the cycle is self-demoralization. Not only do abusers put victims down, but victims also begin to behave in ways that abolish self-respect. They may lie to protect abusers, or helplessly watch as others are abused. Victims at this stage suffer a devastating loss of self-respect and feelings of depersonalization (separation of self from the situation and from their own emotions). They experience guilt and a shattered sense of personal values and belonging, resulting in diminished self-worth and withdrawal from activities. The cycle repeats, as hyperalert victims with low self-esteem will now do anything to please abusers and avoid the abuse.

Lee listened and then said, "It's so obvious now that my interpretation of events as a child influenced my actions as a wife. I believed that if I were *good* and took care of others, all would be well. But all was not well; I was just hiding—perhaps to stay alive. I hid at eight and at thirty, and I continue to hide today. I hid behind my role as the 'good one.' Complying, keeping the peace, making all happy, these are my roles. I now realize without *my* role, there is no cycle."

As Lee reinterpreted her past, she shared new thoughts: "My coping mechanisms were all I had; they served me well, but I no longer need them. I no longer believe that I am bad, nor that I should protect others at my own expense. I feel angry that I was not cared for, and uncomfortable, as I have not previously allowed myself to feel. All this time I believed I was the one who had to change. Letting go of this pressure to please others feels freeing, and I am excited to please me." I congratulate Lee on her intense reflection and for being the fastest learner I had known.

*Reflection* has been defined as an "expertise-enhancing metacognitive, tacit process whereby personal experience informs practice."[121] Others have defined *critical reflection* as an "active interior state that uses cognitive, affective, imaginative and creative means to perceive, represent in language and thereby undergo one's lived experience."[122] Put simply, reflection is a personal thought process that allows us to look inward and make meaning of our lives. Self-reflection is the process of *metathinking*, or thinking about one's own thoughts. In doing that, we discover ourselves. Reflective practice is defined by the psychologist Dr. Elizabeth Boyd as "the process of examining an experience that raises an issue of concern, as an internal process that individuals use to help refine their understanding of an experience, which may lead to changes in their perspectives."[123]

Lack of self-reflection prevents us from observing gaps in ourselves, and as a result we remain at risk for repeating patterns of behaviors that contribute to poor health, ineffective relationships, suboptimal performance, and burnout. The absence of reflection limits our ability to function optimally and reach our full potential. Organizations, like individuals, require reflection; an institution's inability to be reflective and learn from its mistakes limits its ability to improve or reach its potential.[50] By reflecting, we reconstruct events and reprocess experiences to attain a deeper understanding of both the objective occurrences and our human tendency for subjective interpretation.

Reflection is enhanced by, and enhances, narrative writing. Writing is a means of assessing one's ability to reflect, and it is also a "means of attaining the state of reflection."[121,122] Richard Miller, narrative theorist and author of *Writing at the End of the World*, describes writing as "not a solo act."[124] Putting a narrative story to pen and paper brings the invisible to sight for both the self and observers and also gives readers the power to validate, deny, judge, support, praise, or criticize.

Personal reflection and storytelling have been introduced into medical education to serve many purposes, and their value is recognized under numerous competencies defined by the Accreditation Council for Graduate Medical Education in its outcomes project.[121,122,125,126] First, the power of obtaining patients' stories allows students and health-care providers a deeper understanding of patients' experiences, resulting in a rich appreciation of their illnesses and a greater ability to empathize with and advocate for them. Professionals can effectively teach and learn by prompting patients to piece together the context in which their health and life have occurred. Second, it provides future physicians the same ability to understand and appreciate their own life experiences. Entering medicine, many medical students are naive about the culture and have difficulty coping. Without understanding their journey, they become at risk for developing the poor health habits, burnout, depression, and suicide experienced by many in the profession.[51] Third, reflective writing allows for self-assessment of competency. Learners trained in self-reflection can self-direct their learning. Last, reflective writing supports basic written and oral communication skills, which are critically necessary in medicine. As Dr. Rita Charon, director of Columbia University's program in narrative writing says, "Our deepening sense of story will open us to the vastness, the lostness, the uncertainty, and the meanings that unite all who are ill and all of us who do our best to care for them."[122]

As I drove home that evening, I thought about how until I reached the age of forty, reflection seemed counterproductive to my goals of doing. Surrounded by high-achieving parents, mentors, and colleagues, I was taught that action mattered, and I found no value in, or time for, reflecting on my actions. It would take my being overwhelmed and ineffective to discover the power of personal writing and reflection.

I have learned that the busier I am, the more time I need to reflect. As Saint Francis of Assisi states, "Half an hour's meditation each day is essential, except when you *are busy. Then a full hour is needed.*"[127] Going inward allows me to appreciate what Jon Kabat-Zinn calls "non-doing" as critical to my health.[128] Years after my mother asked, "Is medicine really what you want to do?" she again observed me at my worst trying unsuccessfully to manage a clinical practice, teach medical students, direct a research team, and raise two daughters. "How can anyone do all that?" she asked. I acknowledged that I was burning out and paradoxically discovered that less is more. I realized I could do anything but not everything. I learned to value reflection time equal to my time for other tasks and began to block out time for it on my calendar. I now reflect daily in my journal, particularly focusing on areas where I am not getting the results I hoped for. I also choose a "word of the year": rereading my last year's journal, I choose a word that summarizes my learnings. I put the word on the cover of my next journal, in my wallet, and on a sticky note on my laptop. The first word I chose was *present*, to reflect my state of being mindful, the moment of time between past and future, and the gift I give to myself in reflecting. Reflective writing has guided me to create space, grow personally, redefine success, and sustain my health. Experiences serve as prompts for my writing, and writing prompts comprehension of my experiences. As I reflect on journaling, I am grateful for the space created by writing to know myself.

## November 2013–June 2014

Despite Lee's insights, she continued to have ambivalence about her relationship. Her marriage seemed strong one month and at its breaking point the next. Sarah, WISE experts, and I worked regularly with Lee, listening, reflecting her ambivalence, validating her fears, minimizing her isolation, and offering resources. Lee repeatedly said how much she loved her husband and wanted to have a strong family. WISE arranged for Lee to meet women with similar stories. We made calls to Lee's daughter, provided safety plans, and helped Lee hide keys, money, and plane tickets for emergency use. Every visit, Lee convinced herself she could save her family and her marriage. She never gave up hope; we never gave up hope.

Martin and Lee's relationship was not atypical. The National Intimate Partner and Sexual Violence Survey reports that one person in four experiences domestic violence in her lifetime, and the majority of the victims are female. Most cases never get reported to the police. One-third of female homicide victims are killed by an intimate partner.[129] My role, I told Sarah, was to empower Lee to explore all her options and consider her safety first and foremost. I confessed that I would love it if patients like Lee would just leave. But I remind myself that I can narrate only my own story and Lee must narrate hers.

A few months later Lee shared that the night before she had read a WISE brochure and had seen herself in every story. She had thought about Martin's intolerance of her and her tolerance of him and felt a scream deep within her that no one else could hear. Lee surprised us when she announced, "I am being humiliated and controlled. I don't deserve it."

Having long waited for this moment, I eagerly reflected her words back to her. "You don't deserve it."

She repeated, "I don't deserve it."

We went back and forth repeating her discovery. Lee was like a child having just written her name for the first time. Rereading her journal, she reflected that writing her story had allowed her to see she was in an "abusive relationship."

## Summer 2014

A month prior to her missed appointment, Lee acknowledged for the first time that she might be better off without Martin. She spoke of her fear of being alone but also reflected that she was already alone. She quoted Sequiche Coming Leer: "The death of fear is in doing what you fear to do." She said that his words released her from her fear. She recited the Ojibwa prayer, asking the Sacred One to teach her honor so that she might change and heal. Lee was new that day; she was alive. She contemplated her options: standing up to him, leaving him, moving away, running away. I listened as she proposed a plethora of action plans. I was thrilled that she had made so much progress.

*But had she?* I asked myself, while waiting anxiously to hear back from her. On Wednesday morning I arrived at the office under dark storm clouds to find a voice mail from Lee's daughter, Frances. "Yes, Lee is in Arizona, staying with us." Her message was calm and casual. A second voice mail followed from Lee, her voice shaky: "Martin said you called. I am so sorry for missing my appointment. I'm in Arizona and will be back in Vermont next week. I will reschedule and see you soon." I replayed the message and exhaled. "Lee is alive," I exclaimed out loud and sent an email to Sarah.

A week later Lee was on my schedule. Lee's cheeks were flushed to match her soft pink sweater set. She wore a matching silk scarf, baby blue and pink, tied in a perfect knot. She placed her blood-pressure log and a clay pot of sopaipilla, Native American sweet bread, on my desk. "We're moving," she announced, touching her silver bear necklace.

"We?" I asked.

"Yes, we," she beamed. "I made up my mind. By journaling I realized I was running from one abuser to another and decided it was time for me to stop and to go home. I was confident after looking inward that this was right for me, and I rehearsed my conversation with Martin in my head for days." Lee took a deep breath. "I told Martin I was moving back to Arizona, and he could come if he wished." She feared Martin would manipulate her to change her mind and described how he patronized her by saying, "Sure, someday we can move." For her it was time, and she declared that she was leaving that day to begin looking at real estate. She had a flight already scheduled and would stay temporarily with Frances.

Lee was radiant with pride. She shared how she had gone to Arizona and fallen in love with a small adobe-style home only one mile from Frances and complete with a cactus garden. She felt terrified and elated and couldn't believe she was going home. She had been shocked and relieved when Martin decided to join her. She was a new person and believed being so would change their relationship. Lee thanked me for encouraging her to write her story. Holding her soft, fragile hand, I fought back tears. Sarah's dark-brown eyes searched for reassurance before welling up. Lee's tears also flowed, and the three of us hugged, unsure of the next chapter in Lee's story.

Lee walked out the door just before Sarah's words exploded, "I don't get it. I thought we wanted her to leave him. Why is he going too? Nothing will change! Doesn't she know that? Can't you stop her?"

I reflected on all that I had learned from Lee. "You may be right," I said to Sarah. "This may not be what you or I would choose for Lee, but this is her story and what she has chosen for herself. We have only the privilege of listening and guiding." I embraced Sarah, feeling her exhaustion and knowing she and I would both need time to reflect and write our own stories.

• ✹ • ✷ ▸ • • • • ✹ ◦ •

HEALTH CHALLENGE #4    Practice Self-Reflection, and Keep a Journal

Keeping a journal is like taking good care of your heart.

TED KOSSER

Give yourself the gift of a journal, and write your story. Set aside ten minutes a day to write about your life.

1.  Describe critical experiences that occurred in your life. Let each entry reflect a crucible occurrence, major event, phase, or critical point. Describe the facts and details of how you interpreted the situation.

2. Identify general beliefs that you accepted as truths as a result of your experience(s). What specific and predominant thoughts followed that experience? Be conscious, and observe what your inner voice repeatedly tells you. Write about your behaviors. What feelings and actions are you displaying currently, and how have they been shaped by these thoughts and beliefs?

3. Declare a "word of the year." Reflecting on your journal entries, choose a word that triggers your being mindful of what you have learned about yourself and what you wish to focus on, going forward.

# PART TWO SELF-CARE

. . . . . . . . . . . .

Love yourself first, and everything else falls in line.
LUCILLE BALL

Self-care is the active process of prioritizing personal wellness.
Caring for self is a prerequisite to caring for others. Self-care begins
with self-awareness, includes attention to basic physiological needs,
and concludes with optimal health or the need for self-improvement.

• ✦ ● ● ▶ ● ● ● ● ● ● ●

# FILL YOUR OWN TANK

*Self-compassion is simply giving the same kindness to ourselves
that we would give to others.*

CHRISTOPHER GERMER

Kenny is a forty-five-year-old nurse who cares for others 24-7. He works full-time during the day at the VA hospital on the dialysis unit and evenings seven days a week as a home-health nurse, caring for three to four additional patients a day in their homes. He advocates strongly for each patient, and doctors are grateful to have him on their team. Kenny has won the Nurse of the Year Award on multiple occasions and views his work as a privilege. He takes great pride in serving others and knows he provides the best care possible. As a home-health nurse, he follows homebound patients, many of whom have end-stage diseases of the heart, lungs, and kidneys. He supports them in ways beyond medical care: picking up groceries or bandages, giving them rides, preparing their medications, fixing their meals, and accompanying them to doctor's appointments. He gives patients his cell-phone number and tells them to call him for anything. He checks on patients even after they're discharged from his program. Kenny plays a critical role in his patient's lives, and they do the same in his.

Kenny lives alone in a small house, not far from where he grew up. He describes his home as "scantly decorated, simple, and clean." His kitchen is fully stocked with ready-to-go foods, as cooking is neither an interest nor a priority. He leaves his house before breakfast and grabs takeout on the road. His one home-cooked meal a week is at his mother's home every Sunday, where he spends time with his family after completing patient rounds. Kenny's father died of a heart attack in his early fifties, as did his father's two brothers and sister. Kenny was twenty-five at that time, and he assumed the role of "man of the house," responsible for his younger brothers and sisters. Kenny prides himself on raising his family as his father would have. His siblings are now all married with children, but they still live locally and join him most Sundays for dinner.

Kenny is single and reports being too busy for a second family. He also claims to be too busy to take a vacation, but he rents the same beach house his father previously rented every August for his siblings' families to enjoy. Kenny rarely joins them, with the excuse that he dislikes the heat, the sand, and the sun and that he has no one to cover his patients and doesn't want to inconvenience colleagues.

Kenny is African American and suffers from type 2 diabetes, hypertension, high cholesterol, and obesity. African Americans have the highest overall mortality rate from coronary heart disease of any ethnic group in the United States.[130] They also have a greater incidence of hypertension, heart disease, diabetes, stroke, and kidney disease than people of other races.[131] Contributing factors are not fully understood, but in addition to a delay in the recognition and treatment of high-risk individuals and limited access to cardiovascular care, as much as 50 percent of the increased prevalence can be explained by behaviors that are modifiable.[130,132] Minimizing cardiovascular morbidity and mortality in this population must comprise identification and aggressive treatment of obesity, smoking, elevated blood pressure, diabetes, and elevated lipids.[133]

Kenny's last weight was 302 pounds, his height is six feet, and his body mass index (BMI) is 41. He has been a patient of mine for more than ten years and follows up reluctantly and sporadically. He arrived one afternoon with his can of Classic Coke, declined my nurse's attempt to weigh him, and jokingly admitted failure as I walked in the door. He asked about my family, and me, pleasantly avoiding my questions.

"How are you?" I asked.

"Busy," he replied.

"How are you doing with your goals? Your exercise efforts?"

"Too busy." He smiled.

"How about your diet, any success there?"

"Too busy." He laughed.

He checked his phone. "I can't stay long. Ms. Stewart needs a ride to her cardiologist, Mrs. Rampart's wound is worse, and Mr. Roger needs me to pick up his medications."

"Any time for you?" I asked.

"Too busy."

We both see the irony in our conversation, which has gone on with little variation for years. He has made progress from time to time. His weight fluctuates, with a low of 250 three years ago and a high of 315 just six months ago. On most visits he confesses, "I've been fat all my life; can't change that and it doesn't matter. I keep busy focusing on what matters." I remind him of past successes and how he quit drinking Coke and walked daily when first diagnosed with diabetes two years ago.

At that time his blood sugar was 320, and he was scared. He never said as much, but his behavior was telling. For about six months he asked to be seen regularly, saying he wanted "big sister watching." During that time we partnered well and set and achieved specific goals. I coached him to identify top priorities, monitor his progress, and celebrate his smallest of successes. I saw his owning his health goals as major progress. He walked a mile every day before work, and at night he packed lunch and healthy snacks to take to work. He checked his weight and blood sugars and kept a log of his progress. He came in monthly "to be held accountable," and together we discussed his challenges and cheered his achievements. He lost more than fifty pounds, but over the next two years he put it all back on. Sunday visits to his mother got less frequent when she greeted him with "You don't look like you've lost any weight. Don't you know, you won't be any help to us if you're dead?"

Like many patients, Kenny remained intermittently motivated. Like many health professionals, Kenny denied that risks applied to him. He often quit before he succeeded and fell into the trap of talking himself out of trying. "Been there, done that" was one of his most famous quotes. Knowing that only he could change himself, I often asked, "What do you think would work for you?" When he wasn't "too busy," he tried new options, and we kept a running list of his efforts and his outcomes.

- Joined Weight Watchers—"don't like group meetings"
- Met with dietician—"no new information"

- Counted calories—"too time consuming"
- Purchased NutriSystem—"bad tasting, waste of money"
- Joined the gym—"uncomfortable in coed environment"
- Hired personal coach—"too expensive"
- Took group exercise classes—"inconvenient"
- Worked out to videotapes at home—"too tired"
- Considered surgery—"too much risk"
- Started Atkins diet—"craved carbs"
- Walked at work—"no time for breaks and can't shower"
- Tried the Mediterranean diet—"no time to shop or to cook"
- Considered weight-loss medication—"too many side effects"

I was always excited to provide resources when he agreed to try again, knowing different options worked for different people at different times. I shared data and stories of success from other patients. I remained optimistic, cheering Kenny on, but often felt he agreed to options more for me than for himself.

## The Obesity Epidemic

Obesity is a worldwide health concern affecting more than one in every three adults in the United States. A major risk factor for cardiovascular disease and the leading cause of death, obesity is associated with increased mortality and numerous health problems, including hypertension, high cholesterol, diabetes, cancers, musculoskeletal problems, sleep apnea, depression, and infertility.[134] In children and adolescents, obesity is strongly associated with increased cardiovascular mortality in adulthood.[135] In addition to causing physical harms in overweight individuals, obesity affects emotional health. In a culture that values the "perfect body," obesity carries a great social stigma. Women with higher BMIs have lower wages and experience workplace discrimination, contributing to a higher risk of depression and low self-esteem.[136]

Maintaining an ideal body weight is essential for everyone. The U.S. Preventive Services Task Force recommends screening all adults for obesity.[137] BMI is a measure of body fat based on height and weight. A measurement in the range of 20–25 is "normal," 25–29 is "overweight," 30–39 is considered "obesity," and above 40 is considered "extreme obesity." Not only are the rates of obesity increasing, but the rates of extreme obesity also rose 70 percent between 2000 and 2010, going from 3.9 to 6.6 percent of the population.[138] Causes of the obesity epidemic include access to and frequency of eating high-fat and high-sugar food, as well as growing tendencies to lead a sedentary lifestyle. Americans report that 40 percent of their meals are eaten out, and one American in four visits a fast-food restaurant daily.

## The Science of Healthy Eating and Exercise

The cornerstone of prevention and treatment of obesity is lifestyle change. Changes primarily include regular exercise and healthy eating.[139,140] There is strong evidence that basics like a balanced diet, adequate sleep, and daily exercise reduce risks for obesity. Exercise and diet are important for everyone, but they are particularly critical for those with elevated BMI, as even modest amounts of weight loss have been associated with reduced health problems. Committing to healthy food choices as habitually as brushing your teeth prevents negative health consequences.

The care of patients with obesity is complex, even though the science of weight loss is simple. A comprehensive weight-loss program that includes personal behavioral change in partnership with a primary-care physician and team can be very effective for those with elevated BMI.[141] The ultimate goal is to create a daily energy deficit. For every 3,500 calories reduced, one pound is lost. Reducing 500 calories per day over seven days, while not easy, will result in a one-pound loss weekly. Every five pounds lost translates to a one-point reduction in BMI. Calories can be cut by reducing intake (diet) or by increasing utilization (exercise). A realistic goal is a 10 percent weight reduction over a six-month period.

Many diets are available; three examples for which evidence supports their benefits to health are the Dietary Approaches to Stop Hypertension (DASH) eating plan, the Mediterranean diet, and a low-carbohydrate and high-protein diet, such as the Paleolithic or Atkins.[142-146] All three diets eliminate a need for calorie counting, as they rely on diminished appetite coupled with a strong commitment to embracing a new and healthy lifestyle that follows reduced carbohydrates.

The American Health Association states that increasing exercise at any age, by any level, reduces cardiovascular risks. Exercise has been shown to decrease depression in all patients and to benefit caregivers of patients with cancer.[147] Specific adult recommendations include at least 150 minutes of moderately intense aerobic exercise or 75 minutes of vigorous exercise weekly, and muscle-strengthening activities for all muscle groups at least twice per week. Most adults can achieve this with a 30-minute commitment to exercise daily.

## The Life-Changing Event

Two months later, in my office, I was not surprised to receive a note from the cardiologist saying that Kenny was hospitalized. A week later he was in my office; a bottle of water replaced his usual can of Coke, and he willingly allowed my nurse to weigh him. He made no jokes, no inquiry of my family, and no excuse of being busy. As I walked in, he reported his information as if it belonged to one of his patients.

A week ago he was lifting Mr. Turner out of his bed. He experienced pain in his back and chest but wrote it off as a pulled muscle. The next day it returned while he was guiding another patient up the stairs. He ignored it. Two days later the pain returned in the hospital parking lot, while he was leaving his shift to go do home care. It lasted fifteen minutes, and a co-worker who was walking with him insisted that he go to the emergency department.

He arrived that evening in the emergency room winded and shaky. His EKG showed ST segment depression and prominent T-wave inversion in leads $V_5$–$V_6$. He knew that these changes were indicative of ischemia to the lateral aspect of his heart (reduced oxygen to his left heart muscle), probable occlusion of the circumflex coronary vessel (a narrowing of a main blood vessel to his heart), thrombus in the lumen (a blood clot blocking the blood vessel), and likely myocardial infarction (a heart attack). He had read the report himself as it was being generated. The emergency-room doctor, who knew him, said, "You were lucky. This time."

Before Kenny left the emergency room, the bariatric surgery team was consulted and gave him information on the procedure and possible short- and long-term outcomes. He was told that the overall risk of dying from bariatric surgery was less than 0.5 percent (one of every two hundred), but patients like him, who were obese and diabetic, had a higher risk of death. The surgery, he was told, reduced all-cause mortality by 30–50 percent after between seven and fifteen years. In patients with diabetes, 60 percent experience remission, and 30 percent remain without signs of diabetes fifteen years after the procedure.[148] He was told that his weight and health conditions made him eligible for the procedure but that he needed to complete a comprehensive evaluation, including lab work, studies, informational meetings, and online educational seminars, before he could meet the surgeon or be scheduled for the surgery.

Kenny sat in my office, denying any further pain but admitting that he was scared. "I don't like being the patient." He stated that his heart attack was an unwelcome wake-up call. He admitted that he preferred being the nurse and focusing on the health of others. He felt lost being out of work, having so much time to focus on himself. He hesitated, saying, "I guess I should take better care of me if I want to stay around. I don't know what to do. I am afraid of bariatric surgery, but I am not sure I can lose the weight on my own."

It was during this time I spent with Kenny that I reflected on what I have learned about self-care: caring for myself has been helpful in caring for others like Kenny. I hoped that Kenny could take advantage of his fear and make changes, as he had done with his diabetes. I shared Kenny's satisfaction in seeing others succeed, but, unlike him, I was also conscious that my own health is what allows me to support others.

Over the next six months Kenny's fear was sustained, and his motivation grew. He saw me regularly and underwent extensive preparation for bariatric surgery. Again we set specific and achievable goals. He met with a dietician, drastically changed his eating habits, and took thirty-minute walks every morning. He lost 10 percent of his weight (thirty pounds) and made a difficult decision to return only to his work as a visiting nurse. He gave up his hospital job, acknowledging that home care was where he was most needed, and it gave him flexibility and time for himself. Kenny attended group information meetings, talked to patients who had undergone the surgery, and attended personal therapy. He completed the online seminar and all the testing to assess his physical, emotional, mental, and social supports. The Roux-en-y gastric bypass procedure was specifically recommended to him because of its success in patients with extreme obesity and diabetes. He was scheduled with the surgeon to discuss surgery details as well as the follow-up and supplements required after the procedure.

Kenny's next visit with me was a preoperative exam. He shared that he was having second thoughts, not because of the risks of the surgery but for fear of failing his family and friends. His siblings, who were all obese, were supportive and watching. His patients, who struggled with chronic disease, many who were obese, were also cheering for him. His mother had abstained from negative comments at Sunday dinner and altered their meals on the basis of his dietician's recommendations. He was ambivalent because he feared a failure on his part would negatively affect others. Sitting across from me in the office, sweating profusely and struggling to fit comfortably across two chairs, Kenny asked, "What would you do?"

I shared that I had mixed feelings on the value of bariatric surgery. Initially a skeptic, I feared patients would choose it as a quick fix and not change their behaviors. But the data supporting sustainable weight loss are stronger with surgery than with other diet programs, and my experiences with patients had been mostly positive. I have seen patients successfully commit to working hard and really transform themselves. But without an authentic commitment to themselves, patients revert to prior habits of poor eating, sedentary lifestyles, and self-destructive thoughts. I have seen past failure beat down on even those most desperate for change. Success is necessary to fuel further success but does not always overcome negative thinking. A patient of mine, Katie, succeeded at losing weight after surgery but still saw herself as worthless. She continued to criticize herself, gained back the weight, and declared herself a failure. Another patient, Kathleen, worked just as hard on her self-esteem as she did on her weight and ultimately gave herself a new life. She committed fully to personal success and adopted a mantra of "I matter." I shared with Kenny that I thought powerful transformation was possible as a result of surgery, which to its credit requires a holistic look at weight in the context of health and life. Surgical candidates forced to face their strengths and weaknesses can change their lives. I told Kenny that the surgery he faced was not the greatest risk to his health; the greatest risk was not caring for himself.

Drinking his bottle of water, Kenny adjusted his seat and asked, "What should I do?"

My advice to Kenny was to "fill your own tank first." I suggested to him that maximizing his own capacity would contribute to others. I told Kenny, "Self-care is simple, but not easy. You have spent so much time looking at others' needs; this will feel foreign and require refocusing and acknowledging that *you* matter. You can do this. You have the knowledge. Your only weakness is in not applying it to yourself. Look at your opportunity. The process of becoming eligible for surgery is meant to test you. What you think, feel, and do will influence your success. By understanding and acknowledging why you have not previously cared for yourself, you can begin to change your behaviors and your life."

"I know I'm not invincible and the risks apply to me. So is it that I don't care about me?" Kenny wondered. "That I don't care about my own health? Is it that I don't believe I matter, or . . . ?" Contemplating bariatric surgery provided Kenny an opportunity to see his ambivalence. He acknowledged he wanted to care for his family, his patients, and himself. He realized that he couldn't wait until he was done caring for others to focus on himself. He ended this presurgery visit acknowledging he had a lot to think about and asking himself one last question: "Can I change?"

## No One Is Immune

There remains a question as to the effectiveness and capabilities of health professionals, who are reported as 40 percent overweight and 6 percent obese, to counsel patients in areas where they themselves struggle.[149,150,151] Using the "tank full" metaphor, I scan and monitor my own health regularly. I haven't always practiced self-care, and like Kenny I once believed being a provider meant my purpose was to focus on caring for others. I have learned that when I am well, I can fully give to others, but when I am not, I must address my own needs first. As a resident in family medicine, I trained under Dr. Clive Brock, a physician from South Africa and an international expert in Balint training.[152] Dr. Michael Balint was a British psychiatrist who coined the phrase "doctor as the pill." He believed the power of physicians to heal comes from their ability to fully commit to the patient-doctor relationship, to engage patients as people, and to actively listen, not just to dispense medication. Dr. Brock taught me that "prescribing medication is often necessary but never sufficient." He encouraged us as residents to balance our role in giving with our role in addressing our own needs. He believed that within the patient-doctor relationship both parties' health mattered. He taught that what I gave depended on how much I had to give, not only in the form of pills from my black bag but in the giving of my own eyes, ears, mouth, and heart.

In residency I struggled to achieve balance in health and in life. My exercise was limited to walking across hospital floors, and I kept my blood sugar from falling in the middle of the night by drinking cans of Ensure in elevators between admissions. Dr. Brock taught me that no one is immune to imbalance and that I am equally vulnerable and as much in need of personal health and wellness as my patients. I came to appreciate how fundamental my personal health was to my success as a doctor. No matter what my task, my own health must be tended to first. In my journal, where I keep my values, purpose, and vision, I now scan my health. I set yearlong goals and list them on the back cover to review regularly. My goals vary each year, but over the past decade many, such as those focused on eating, sleeping, and exercising, remain constant. My journal is a powerful reminder to assess and fill my tank. With each goal I set and achieve, I trust myself to prioritize me.

Over the years I have observed colleagues struggling to maintain balance and health, in numbers equal to the patients who were doing so. The need is most evident in physical health, with many reporting eating unhealthy meals on the run, being overweight, forgoing regular exercise, and being chronically tired. It is also apparent in emotional health, with their rampant negativity and diminished volunteering, and a great number acknowledge being worn out and disengaged. Just like shoemakers who wear no shoes, when health professionals ignore their own needs, they become vulnerable: the cardiologist who is morbidly obese, the oncologist who smokes, the family physician who is stressed. As a consultant on personal wellness and improvement in health-care settings across the globe, I see health professionals as among the last to consider their own health needs. I am disappointed to find burnout also on the rise in Eastern cultures, as it is in the West, but I am hopeful, given the growing requests for training in personal health improvement across systems, disciplines, and professions.

A nurse who attended one of my workshops raised her hand to ask fellow attendees the obvious: "How can we ask our patients to do what we say but not what we do?" My workshop objectives included discussing strategies that health professionals apply to themselves to sustain health and prevent burnout. The irony, in my experience, is that strategies shared by health professionals often come from their patients, and in the course of that sharing are passed back to their patients. Medicine is an apprenticeship model, and faculty behaviors are modeled and often become the behaviors of learners. Self-care is particularly critical for aspiring professionals who enter a culture where they perceive a need for permission to actively pursue their own health. A resident I taught shared that when he arrived as a new first-year student, he discontinued his practice of walking every afternoon while listening to medical journals on audiotapes, for fear of being viewed as "not working hard enough." Instead, he sat in his office, with the door closed, feeling resentful and alone. He reminded me that we are all patients, and, as such, our health matters.

## The Power of Self-Care

In the end, Kenny fully committed to caring for himself and was steadfast in doing so *without* bariatric surgery. Over eighteen months he lost more than a hundred pounds. He achieved a long-awaited goal of dropping below two hundred pounds, gaining enormous insight in the course of his journey. He described a newfound power to serve others, and he honored me by claiming that his personal success came from "filling his own tank first." We tapered him off all medications for diabetes. He no longer experiences chest pain. He is going strong with his exercise goal and gets his daily fruits and vegetables.

Whenever I have a student with me during his visit, I ask Kenny to share what he learned on his journey. Never hesitating, he recites from his long list of learnings:

1. I always make sure to eat breakfast.
2. I remember that self-neglect has many faces and many voices and that the main concept, no matter what my excuses, is that my health matters.
3. Fear is a great motivator.
4. My purpose has to always include caring for me, or I won't be here to achieve it.

5. Eating healthily and exercising is hard, but I feel so good, I don't think I could ever stop.
6. I have so much energy.
7. Self-image is linked to self-care, and insecurities and poor ego come from the lack of trusting me.
8. With each small success, I begin to believe in myself, and I break past cycles of failure.
9. I am proud of myself.
10. I really am a healthy role model, which allows me to give more genuinely to others.
11. Taking care of my health beats the alternative.

Kenny has had success equal to that of any bariatric surgery patient, and I trust he will sustain his efforts, as he now believes that his health matters. He deserves full credit for his success and for the success of those who have benefited from his efforts. Self-care is not a weakness but a sign of personal strength, commitment, and success. Both he and I now know that by filling our own tanks, we not only benefit personally but also advance our ability to care for others. Prioritizing our personal health sets the example, giving others permission to do the same. I am proud of myself and of Kenny, and I know the well-being and sustainability of our population depends on, and is determined by, the health of each of us.

•  ✎  ●  ➤   ●  ●  ●  ●  ✎  ▲  ▫

HEALTH CHALLENGE #5     Nourish Your Body, Mind, and Spirit

The most powerful relationship you will ever have is the relationship with yourself.
STEVE MARABOLI

Review the health behaviors worksheet below to assess your degree of holistic self-care and your readiness to make changes when needed. In lesson 9 you will have the opportunity to prioritize and improve a specific area of your health. Consider healthy eating and exercise if you have not already succeeded in these fundamental areas. Calculate your BMI. Is it greater than 25? If so, set up an appointment with your primary-care physician and make

# HEALTH BEHAVIOR WORKSHEET

| | MY RESPONSE (check appropriate column) | | MY READINESS TO CHANGE* | | |
|---|---|---|---|---|---|
| | Agree | Disagree | | | |
| I have healthy eating habits. | | | 1 | 2 | 3 |
| I exercise regularly. | | | 1 | 2 | 3 |
| I am at or near my ideal body weight and am happy with my body image. | | | 1 | 2 | 3 |
| I get sufficient sleep. | | | 1 | 2 | 3 |
| I do not use tobacco products. | | | 1 | 2 | 3 |
| I drink alcohol less than: fourteen drinks per week (men), or seven drinks per week (women). | | | 1 | 2 | 3 |
| I always put on my seat belt. | | | 1 | 2 | 3 |
| I always wear a helmet when cycling. | | | 1 | 2 | 3 |
| If I keep firearms, they are stored unloaded and locked up. | | | 1 | 2 | 3 |
| If I am sexually active with multiple partners, I use contraceptives and practice safe sex every time. | | | 1 | 2 | 3 |
| I receive routine recommended health-care screenings and vaccines as appropriate. | | | 1 | 2 | 3 |
| I often wash my hands (and always before eating). | | | 1 | 2 | 3 |
| I use required prescription drugs appropriately. | | | 1 | 2 | 3 |
| I do not use illegal drugs. | | | 1 | 2 | 3 |
| I am safe with my partner and comfortable with how we work out our differences. | | | 1 | 2 | 3 |
| I take time off when I am sick. | | | 1 | 2 | 3 |
| I have time alone for mindful meditation and reflection. | | | 1 | 2 | 3 |
| I cope with stress in healthy and effective ways. | | | 1 | 2 | 3 |
| I manage my time and balance my workload effectively. | | | 1 | 2 | 3 |
| I am balanced in my use of electronics. | | | 1 | 2 | 3 |
| I express my emotions as they come and in healthy ways. | | | 1 | 2 | 3 |
| I affirm my value and purpose regularly. | | | 1 | 2 | 3 |
| I spend time with supportive friends and family. | | | 1 | 2 | 3 |
| I prioritize spending on things that support my health. | | | 1 | 2 | 3 |
| Other behavior(s) I wish to change include: | | | 1 | 2 | 3 |

*1 = ready to change; 2 = thinking about change; 3 = not thinking about change a weight management plan. Many additional formal tools and surveys exist for individuals to assess their own health status, including an easy-to-use and free site, HowsYourHealth.org, developed by John Wasson, MD, emeritus professor at Dartmouth's medical school and licensed by the Trustees of Dartmouth College.

● ● ● ● ● ● ● ● ● ● ●

# ESTABLISH TRUSTING RELATIONSHIPS

*I travel to many places around the world, and whenever I speak to people,*
*I do so with the feeling that I am a member of their own family.*
THE DALAI LAMA

## The Day Embedded in Ink

When I first met Christina, it was mid-June 2014. She told my nurse she was there for antibiotics and nothing more. She was scheduled for twenty minutes, refused to see my medical student, and stood next to the door when I entered. Christina averted her eyes, remained standing, and abruptly described a headache, fever, and cold that had persisted over the past month despite her quitting smoking last week. Sensing her desire for space, I allowed her to continue, offering only congratulations on quitting. I apologized for the intrusion of my computer and glanced briefly at her nearly empty medical record. Her eyes were still averted as I examined her. I was struck by the I-don't-care attitude written across her face and the multitude of tattoos covering much of her body. On her neck read, "Life ends 6-18-13." Each limb carried another message. Her left leg read, "DAMAGED." Her right arm read, "PAIN is Strength." Across her chest was a list of names: "Jeremy, Bianca, Eugene." The letters across her back read, "BROKEN." She bore a story in ink, permanently embedded in her skin. As today was June 11, 2014, I ignored my tightly booked clinical schedule and gently opened Pandora's box. I asked about the date, and I asked about the names. Not expecting my questions, she looked up. Her eyes looked into mine for the first time, and tears welled up.

"She was all I had. I loved her; I can't go on. She was all I had, and I failed her. She is no more. She is nothing. Her life is gone and so is mine. She loved me, and now she's gone. She trusted me. No one should trust me. I don't trust myself. They told me I would fail, and I failed. My mother told me not to trust anyone, but I did. I trusted Bianca, and I shouldn't have trusted her. I shouldn't have believed her. I shouldn't have let her lie to me. I told her the world was safe. I lied to her. I wanted to protect her. I didn't protect her. I didn't teach her to protect herself. I didn't say no. I didn't teach Bianca to say No! Now she is gone."

Christina's grief hung in the air, as palpable as her tears. She referred to everything in life as either before or after "The Day." The Day was June 18, 2013. That date was the day that she found Bianca, her eighteen-year-old daughter, dead. Christina described life after that day. Everything stopped. The world felt heavy, then it felt small, and then it was dead. Christina dropped out of life and ceased to participate in anything. She said that after that day she was unable to move, to go to the dentist or to the school PTA, to return to work, or even to read a newspaper. She couldn't talk to family or neighbors; she couldn't leave the house. The weight she carried was too heavy. Christina declined offers of help, not wanting to be lifted. She was relieved to not care, to not trust, and to not rely on anyone. After The Day, she remained alive for the sole purpose of caring for her eight-year-old son, Eugene. She tolerated the rest of the world. She had lost her most precious daughter and visibly wore a tattoo of shame. She labeled herself "broken" and accepted all abandonment and the stigma of society.

I listened while she talked. I recalled my own heaviness the year my oldest daughter left for college. But my loss was softened by my joy at knowing that her dreams and hopes were fully alive. I shuddered at the possibility of my daughter's being gone forever. I felt both empty and saturated with the grief I saw in Christina's bloodshot eyes. I thanked her for sharing, gave her an antibiotic, and invited her to follow up in a week or sooner if the infection didn't resolve. It was not a coincidence that I scheduled her to come back exactly a week later. I wanted to be with her on the anniversary of The Day. Christina was noncommittal but accepted the prescription and the appointment.

As we left the room, my student, Sarah, approached us in the hall. Christina, with a wad of tissues in her hand, stepped aside and stared at Sarah. Sarah has dark-brown eyes, she is small and lean, and her straight brown hair was pulled back in a long ponytail. She wore a scarf wrapped around her neck and a brightly colored, flowing sundress. I introduced them to each other, and Christina's eyes fixed on Sarah's. She reached to shake her hand, whispering, "You look exactly like my Bianca."

One week later, on June 18, Christina appeared on my schedule and reported to the nurse that her headache and cold symptoms were better. She accepted my nurse's offer to have Sarah join me. She held herself together long enough for the nurse to check her blood pressure and weight and to leave the room. When Sarah and I entered, her eyes turned to Sarah, and her tears flowed. I arranged the box of tissues in front of her as her words began to pour forth.

"Living with Bianca was wonderful and horrifying. We did everything together, and then we didn't. We built so many traditions, and then we had none. We danced and we sang. We swore and we cried. She was beautiful, and she was dangerous. She was an angel, and she was the devil himself. She cared and she cuddled and she lied and she stole." Christina sobbed as she spoke. "She was kind and gentle and scary and manipulative. She was home for days and then she was gone, missing for weeks. Then she would appear for meals as if nothing had changed. She asked for money and would go missing again. She stole her father's prescriptions for oxycodone and did worse under my roof." Her sobbing continued, but her words paused. She caught her breath and continued:

One night Bianca went into her bedroom, and the next day she didn't come out. I went in and found her. She looked dead. The ambulance came. They said her heart was still beating, just slowly. They said she was still breathing, just slowly. They said her pupils were small. They were always small. They gave her a shot. She came alive. They said it was an overdose. They asked if she had attempted suicide. They sent her to rehabilitation. Three weeks later she came home. She said she was fine. I believed her. I refused to acknowledge she had a drug problem. I knew it, and I should have stopped it. I should have, but I didn't. It happened again. She was dead and then she was alive, like Lazarus, over and over again. I became numb to her death, grateful and resentful of that resurrecting naloxone shot.

Christina was visibly shaking as she spoke about Bianca, tissues bunched up across her lap. She touched the tattoo on her neck and continued to speak. "On June 18 the ambulance arrived. They said her heart had stopped. They said she wasn't breathing. They gave her the shot. They tried to save her; they gave her another shot; they said she was gone. I stared forever into her small brown eyes; they remained forever small."

## The Opioid Epidemic

Today's opioid epidemic is the worst in our country's history, hitting all regions, and is now being called the greatest threat to our society's health.[153] Deaths from overdoses of heroin and prescription opioids, such as oxycodone, hydrocodone, and methadone, have nearly quadrupled since 1999 and are still rising and destroying families and communities all across our nation. Drug overdose is now the leading cause of injury-related death. In 2014 there were well over twenty-eight thousand deaths from drug overdose in the United States, outnumbering the motor-vehicle fatalities. Rural and suburban areas are some of the hardest hit, with 75 percent of the opiate-addicted population living in those communities. These areas where the economy has been hit disproportionately hard also lack resources for recovery, as the overwhelming majority of treatment centers remain urban. The costs to society for health care and rehabilitation are in the billions.[154,155]

The epidemic that began at the turn of the century has been blamed on many factors, including a push by pharmaceutical companies, medical societies, hospitals, and doctors to alleviate pain with opioids. In 1996 the American Pain Society recommended that doctors consider pain the "fifth vital sign."[156] The intent was largely a commitment to relieve suffering and to overcome physician's reluctance to prescribe pain medication. Many believe this was initiated hastily and without sufficient emphasis on addiction awareness or training. In 2001 the Joint Commission, which accredits health-care organizations, included standards for pain management in a practical guidebook for clinicians, with a statement that "if patients became tolerant to opioid medications the dose could be increased and that doctors need not operate under exaggerated and outdated fears of addiction."[157]

More than half of drug-overdose deaths in 2013 were attributable to prescription opioids or heroin. One person out of every ten who take opioids becomes addicted, and the risk rises in teenagers. Those who become addicted to prescription opioids such as oxycodone may turn to illegal drugs, and those addicted to illegal drugs such as heroine seek prescription drugs to fulfill their addiction. The impact of addiction is powerful and reverberates beyond the addicted individual to entire communities.

Successfully treating pain and addiction requires trusting relationships, but even they offer no guarantees. Strategies and policies exist to require close follow-up, communication, and monitoring of risks and side effects. Contracts serve as tools to clarify expectations and to promote bidirectional trust and respect between patients and physicians. But contracts can be broken, policies ignored, and medications misused. Resources are limited, and patients often move from one practice to another. The U.S. and state attorneys general are working across state lines to ensure that prescription usage and information on trafficking of illegal opioids are being shared. Efforts are also being ramped up to educate the public and health professionals about addiction, emergency and recovery treatment, and overdose medications like naloxone.

## Two Years after The Day

In 2015, two years after Bianca's death, Christina still cried. Sometimes she refused to believe Bianca was gone. Occasionally, she was angry, bargaining with herself, playing the "what if" game. Other times her mood resembled depression, but she had yet to reach a stage of acceptance. She was alone most of her days and spiraled down in her isolation. While her young son, Eugene, was at school, she remained in the house. She didn't sleep well and admitted she didn't know if life was worth living. She denied suicidal thoughts and acknowledged that Eugene was her only reason to live. She refused my recommendations for counseling and medication. She desperately wanted to bring her elder son, Jeremy, back home, but she knew he still used drugs, and she couldn't face thinking she might find him dead as well. Her only progress was in mothering Eugene. She tried hard to keep up their traditions: playing daylong games of Monopoly and Life, having picnics in the living room, and listening to music under the stars before bedtime. Although these activities reminded her of Bianca, she was committed to keeping them going and to honoring her daughter's creative spirit.

During my first few years of practice, I learned that for patients like Christina, my relationship plays a much larger role than for most patients who see me once or twice a year for basic health needs. As a physician, I believe my relationships with all my patients are important, but most people have a network of supports, of which I am one of many contributors. The fewer connections a patient has, the more vulnerable he or she is and the more important my role is. For Christina and others who are secluded for various reasons, I find myself filling a primal human need for communication and connection. Christina comes for visits monthly, and our relationship is often her only adult contact. She is critical of herself and reluctant to see her own strengths. One of my jobs is to acknowledge her successes as a mother and to give her credit for her progress. I felt immense pride after a visit when Christina shared that prior to seeing me, she had avoided all doctors. She said, "I previously felt like a number, but you made me feel like my life and Bianca's life matter, when you first asked about my tattoos and my children." She paused, looked in my eyes, and said, "I felt like you cared. Thank you."

One afternoon Christina appeared on my schedule as an acute visit for "follow-up from a car accident five days prior." Sarah joined us and sat down beside Christina, who reached out to touch Sarah's hand. On the day of the accident, Christina was seen in the emergency room and had gotten X-rays. She was assured nothing was broken and was given ten days' worth of oxycodone for pain and cyclobenzaprine for muscle spasms in her neck and back. She was out of both medications and was in my office to request more. She was adamant that she needed refills and that she couldn't function with the pain. I asked her to describe the pain, to rate the pain, to tell me about her use of ibuprofen, ice, the soft collar, heat, rest, or physical therapy. Christina became irritated, and she declared that nothing else had worked. She declined all my options. She released Sarah's hand and stood up. Visibly agitated, she walked toward the door, saying, "I thought you cared about me. I thought you trusted me. Why won't you treat my pain?"

Sarah's eyes widened as she turned toward me, expecting my answer but seeing only my blank face. In my moment of hesitation, Christina announced she had to use the restroom. She abruptly walked out the door and turned toward the main lobby. I told Sarah what I knew about Christina's life, which had never been easy. Her parents divorced when she was three. Her father was an alcoholic; her mother was in and out of jail on various charges. She was passed around to live with family, abused by their "friends," and introduced to drugs before she was a teenager. Her mother suffered chronic pain, and she recalled how her mother had a steady supply of narcotics as well as drug dealers in whatever house they slept in. She herself was in and out of rehabilitation and dropped out of high school. She was pregnant at sixteen, nineteen, and twenty-nine. She never married any of her children's fathers, as they came and went but could not be relied on for support of any kind. Christina wanted to succeed on her own and protect her children from the childhood that she had experienced. She stayed with friends and family off and on but moved frequently, as her options were often unsafe, time-limited, or not kid-friendly. She herself had only quit using drugs when her oldest son, Jeremy, began using them at the age of twelve.

Christina denied ever feeling connected to her family and struggled to establish friendships. Working off and on cleaning houses and serving fast food, Christina had little time to spend socializing and was always determined to earn enough money to someday own her own house. When her grandmother passed away, she was given her small mobile trailer, where she now lived and which she proudly called home. The only people she remembered ever trusting were her three children. The only person she was currently connected to was eight-year-old Eugene. He needed her, and she wouldn't abandon him.

## Pain, Addiction, and Trust

The heaviness of the situation grew as I recalled Christina's past. I struggled to consider Christina's request for narcotics in the face of her pain, her past addiction, and her relationships. I continued to speak my thoughts to Sarah, to tell her how all three of these issues were core, and all three were entwined in Christina's care. Pain and addiction are two of the most complex maladies to treat, pain being subjective and addiction leaving individuals desperate and vulnerable. Success with both relies heavily on a strong patient-doctor relationship. Honest communication is not always welcome and not easily established in short, rushed visits. Writing a prescription is often quicker than addressing underlying causes of pain or offering alternatives, which can provoke confrontation. Dispensing narcotic prescriptions can be satisfying in the moment but can leave vulnerabilities in the long run.

My decision to prescribe or not to prescribe pain medication to Christina pushed and pulled at the essence of my being a doctor, to alleviate suffering and build trust. I struggled with the delicate balance between benefit and harm that seemed to rest on my prescription pad. I wanted to relieve her pain but not risk supporting an addiction. I knew that she was alone and that she might not come back. I knew she could go elsewhere and potentially get any drugs she wanted. I wished she had allowed a specialist to partner with us. I wished I had insisted on setting up the village to assist in her care. I told Sarah that I was fearful that any decision I made could have a negative impact on Christina's health.

There were many outcomes for Christina. I had seen these far too many times. I cringed as I reflected aloud to Sarah on patients for whom I had prescribed opioids, situations that had resulted in distrust, addiction, arrests, overdose, and even suicide. I feared failing Christina on the multiple levels of pain, addiction, and relationships. Sarah admitted that she had little knowledge about treating pain and no experience with addiction, but she did appreciate the importance of relationships. She shared how hearing my fears and watching me admit to not having the right answer helped her to see the value of sharing her own challenges and fears with others.

I continued to think out loud, piecing together for Sarah and myself what I had learned, hoping to see a best path forward for treating Christina. Patients with pain want relief of pain. Patients with addiction want narcotics. Observing the difference is critical. Most patients with pain don't want or need narcotics. Most patients with pain fear addictive medications. They fear an inability to function; they fear dependence; they fear the side effects of narcotics: the nausea, drowsiness, and constipation. Many are even willing to live in pain to avoid these. Most patients with pain prefer trying anything to avoid using addictive medications regularly.

To accurately diagnose pain, there must be trust, for there is no way to confirm or to disprove its presence. Pain can significantly limit function and destroy a person's will to live. And physical pain is not the only cause of suffering. Those with mental, emotional, and social pain, who are broken, lost, exhausted, and grieving, can be devastated. Pain can be aggravated by and can contribute to stress. Patients who suffer chronic loss can lack the will to function. When life feels purposeless, pain is poorly tolerated. Patients in distress have a lower threshold for pain. I trusted that Christina was in pain. She was already suffering emotionally and socially and was at great risk for suffering physically as well.

Patients with addiction can be defensive and verbally aggressive. Many feel judged and fear getting cut off from their medications. Patients with addiction often refuse to try options other than opioids. Many are willing to give their lives to have these medications. Addiction is a full-time job. It demands full attention to achieve its goal. Patients addicted to prescription drugs are notorious for "doctor shopping." They move around frequently and show up on schedules as new patients who just moved to the area and need refills of their medications.

We as physicians often label patients with addiction as difficult. Providers don't like confrontation and fear that patients will become belligerent and threatening. Many have heard the excuses: the bottle spilled down the drain or was left behind on a trip; the prescription was eaten by the dog, stolen in the car, or dissolved in the washing machine. Many physicians also have experiences that feed their fears: that prescriptions they have written in good faith will be misused, sold, or used to the point of overdose or even death. They fear they will lose their license. Christina had all the red flags and the risks for addiction. Those with past addiction are at risk for future addiction. Treating pain is more difficult in the face of addiction, and addressing addiction is more challenging in the face of pain. In both cases trust and respect are critical.

Relationships are just as important to health as diet and exercise are. Patients with stronger and more diverse relationships are healthier. Isolation has been shown to have negative effects on physical and emotional health in people of all ages. Loneliness and isolation in the elderly has been associated with greater stress, lower immune responses, higher blood pressure, and premature death.[12] The researchers Drs. John and Stephanie Cacioppo found that 40 percent of Americans acknowledge feeling lonely.[10] Patients reporting chronic loneliness had measurably higher stress hormones in the blood and urine and greater fight-or-flight responses, with the full cascade of effects of chronic stress. Adverse health effects have been related to both the length of loneliness and the severity of loneliness.[11] Diverse social networks have long been associated with greater resistance to even the common cold. Sheldon Cohen and colleagues developed the Social Network Index tool to assess participation in twelve types of social relationships and the risk of susceptibility to the common cold. The relationships they looked at included those with a spouse, parents, parents-in-law, children, other close family members, close neighbors, friends, workmates, schoolmates, fellow volunteers, members of groups without religious affiliation, and members of groups focused on religion. The researchers found that susceptibility to colds decreased in a dose-response manner with increased diversity in the social network.[158]

Trusting relationships are important in all aspects of life and are critical in treating pain and addiction. Trust allows for healthy conflict and the expression of diverse opinions without fear of judgment. In a safe environment, the expression of opinion motivates and fosters participation and accountability to ideas and action. Individuals naturally want to trust one another, and, likewise, doctors and patients naturally want to trust each other. When trust is broken, relationships change. Individuals become cautious, guarded, hardened, disengaged, intolerant, and judgmental. Humans are naturally prone to a negativity bias, meaning that negative experiences are more strongly ingrained in our memories than positive experiences. Therefore, broken trust triggers a strong negative experience within a relationship. We are wired to react quickly, activate stress responses, and lay down memories that can direct avoidance and fear of similar future situations. Fear that results from distrust prevents future trust.

As a doctor, I treasure my ability to trust and be trusted. My own experiences in life and with patients have been primarily positive, and I believe in showing trust in others until it proves mistaken. I am, however, conscious of the negative experiences I have had with patients misusing narcotics and realize that these affect my thoughts. I am mindful that my tendency to trust is diminished with patients seeking narcotics, as my thoughts are tainted with fear. With Christina, I dreaded a confrontation that could negate her progress, destroy our relationship, or isolate her further. In negotiating conflict, I have learned that communicating and receiving feedback is difficult, but feedback is a gift. Receiving feedback means someone cares enough about me to observe something that I have done right or wrong and has taken the time to tell me. Giving feedback means I accept that the risk of losing a relationship outweighs the harm of keeping quiet and missing an opportunity to make a difference in someone's life. In the end, my relationship with Christina is what drove my decision, and I hoped it would also allow me to sleep at night without worrying about her safety.

Christina reentered the room. She stood by the door, eyes averted. My palms were sweating, and I struggled with my words, knowing they were not what she wanted to hear. I hoped that she would trust me and trust my decision. "Christina, I care a great deal about you. I know you are suffering. I want you to be happy and to be healthy. I don't want you to struggle, and the last thing I wish to do is to add to your suffering, but I am uncomfortable giving you narcotics for your pain. Giving you narcotics is not in your best interest, and I want you to trust me."

She looked directly into my eyes. Her voice was shaky as her fingers felt across her neck, across the date 6-18-13. "Nothing else works for my pain," she said. "I have tried it all. I need to dull the pain. I need to dull everything. Please just help me."

I steadied my own hand and reached for hers. "Christina, you have been through so much, but you still have much to live for. You have overcome past addiction, but you are vulnerable. You have a beautiful son who needs you. You must move forward with your goals and your life. I want to help you. I believe you have real pain, but narcotics are not our best or only option. They are a last choice for you."

Christina now sat down beside Sarah, who cautiously touched Christina's other hand, just as her tears began to fall.

"I hope that you will not leave my practice. I hope that you will not go to another doctor or seek drugs elsewhere to dull your pain. I hope you will be willing to . . ." I paused.

Tears filled Christina eyes as she spoke. "I don't want to be addicted. I know what I should have done before and what I should have taught Bianca to do. I will 'say no!'" She looked up.

My palms were still sweating as she stood up to leave.

## Three Years after The Day

In June 2016 I was elated that Christina was still arriving regularly for visits. She had completed a course of physical therapy, had started doing yoga, and was turning the corner. By reaching out to her older son, Jeremy, and his girlfriend, both of whom she knew were still using drugs, she found meaning in Bianca's loss. She agreed to meet a psychiatrist partner of mine and was in therapy. She began to write poems and to speak openly about Bianca's tragedy. She spoke aloud of her own loss. She said it helped her to know she was keeping Bianca's spirit alive and, more important, that she might keep someone else alive. She expanded her traditions with Eugene to include a "just say no" game to teach him what she learned, and she permanently embedded "family first" in a tattoo across her cheek. Christina showed me how potent a risk factor isolation is to one's health. From her I learned that trust and feedback are key to preserving relationships and sustaining wellness.

• • • • ▸ • • • • • ▪ ▴ •

HEALTH CHALLENGE #6    Give and Receive Feedback

Don't walk in front of me; I may not follow. Don't walk behind me;
I may not lead. Just walk beside me and be my friend.
ALBERT CAMUS

1. Create a list of those you trust; include the names of those who guide you, challenge you, and provide you with feedback about important issues in a way that enhances your health and wellness.
2. Complete the Social Network Index (www.psy.cmu.edu/~scohen /sni.html) to assess your risk of social isolation. For each of the twelve possible high-contact roles, assign a 0 if you do not have the role and a 1 if you do. The total number of high-contact roles is computed by summing the 0s and 1s. One point is assigned for each type of relationship (possible score of 12) for which you indicate that you spoke (in person or on the phone) to someone at least once every two weeks. A score of 1–3 is considered high-risk, and a score greater than 6 is considered low-risk.

3. When you start your day or do something positive, form an intention to dedicate your energy to someone who has contributed to supporting you.
4. Validate your self-SWOT from lesson 2 by asking someone whom you trust (a mentor, colleague, friend, or family member) to also complete a SWOT of you. Compare the two. Offer to complete a SWOT for them.
5. Write a letter to someone you trust, thanking that person for his or her commitment to you.

• • • ▸ • • • • • ▪ •

# REPLENISH 24-7

It's not enough to be busy, so are the ants.
The question is, what are we busy about?

HENRY DAVID THOREAU

"I'm so tired of not sleeping," Shirley began in a harried manner, as I walked into the office. She looked unusually disheveled: hair unbrushed, eyes swollen, mascara smeared, and clothing wrinkled. "I have not slept at all in three days and not well in months. I can't focus. I can't exercise. I'm eating terribly, and I'm not thinking straight. I just need to sleep. I don't want medication. I just want to function, and I need to be there for my children. I dozed off and nearly crossed the median driving yesterday—would have, if not for my son's screams. I'll be fine if I can just sleep."

This was not the Shirley I had known for years: a woman so put together on all levels, she fitted the definition of health, no matter how you defined it. Shirley exercised, ate healthy foods, took no medications, and managed her mild chronic back pain by staying active playing golf and tennis. I saw her annually for physicals and was always impressed with her ability to be balanced. She took amazing care of herself and found purpose giving to others.

At twenty-four she had married her college sweetheart, Roger, now a local surgeon. At thirty-five, she was the mother of two children in middle school, participated fully in their activities, and vacationed regularly at her second home on Cape Cod. She volunteered in the community, sang in the choir, and wrote for the town newsletter. In past visits she had talked endlessly about her plans to expand the community center, oversee a clothing drive, coordinate a 5K for the hospital, and support urban children coming to summer camp in New Hampshire. She had endless projects, was always busy, and found enormous joy in her life. She was often asked how she had time for everything, and she joked that her initials, sw, stood for Super Woman. The Shirley I knew thrived on having and doing it all.

"What's on your mind and keeping you awake?" I asked, focused on her swollen and bloodshot eyes.

"Roger is having an affair." Shirley's words and tears flooded my office. "I knew," she said, "but I didn't want to know. I hoped it would stop. He hasn't had time for us—in years. He's too busy, as I knew he would be. I saw it coming. I told him so, but he couldn't stop. I don't hate him, but I hate knowing what we are losing. Caring for our family is too much for him, just as it was too much for our fathers. He has no time: for me, for our children, for dinner, or for life. He shut down—he stopped caring." Shirley smoothed her skirt and wiped her eyes.

His work consumes him: his patients, his research, and then his invention thing. He designed some device and wanted to patent it. I don't even know what it does, but it got his time. First, he was excited and shared how he would construct it, then he needed more time to test it, present it, and disseminate it. Then he needed to publish it, and we never saw him. He partnered with colleagues in Boston and was gone every weekend. The more time he spent on it, the less he had for us.

Apparently, Roger was spending weekends at our house on the Cape, and somewhere along the way he met this woman. My sister borrowed our place for a weekend—and they were there. He denies that she means anything to him. The sad part is, I believe him. He can't care about her. How could he? He doesn't even have time to care for himself or for me, and I know he loves me.

Shirley wiped her eyes, more swollen from crying.

For months, I asked myself, what's wrong with him? But now I can't stop thinking, what's wrong with me? I don't matter, and soon I will have nothing and be nothing. All our dreams will be gone. How could we let it happen? When we met in college we were both premed, inspired by our fathers, who were both doctors. We clicked immediately and committed to getting married. We knew the pressure that our family would face, but we promised each other we would give our children more of our time than we got from our parents. After we got married, we agreed that he would continue, but I would postpone medical school to first fulfill my dream of having four children. Roger went on to pursue a residency in surgery, and I focused on our family. We agreed to both do our part to create a more balanced home life than either of us grew up in.

Shirley blew her nose and continued. She said that initially it had worked for them. She did her part and had their first two children in the time it took Roger to rise to the level of an admired attending. But as a stay-at-home parent, she realized early on that she would never leave her children to go to medical school. Initially, Roger came home exhausted but remained engaged. He was excited to share patient stories with the three of them. He gave them elaborate accounts of how he removed stones from Mr. Hardy, saved Mrs. Bundt's life, or removed a tumor from Mr. Bono. He was their hero.

But over the next five years, he became overwhelmed and lost his sense of joy. He rarely made it home for dinner, and they decided two children was plenty. Occasionally, after a second glass of wine, Shirley caught a glimpse of the old Roger, as he spoke of his fear of repeating his father's predictably unreliable patterns. But Roger was a perfectionist, and, even more than imbalance, he feared failure and the stigma of mental illness, believing that "surgeons were "tough." Incapable of appreciating his successes, he focused only on "doing more." He poured himself into work, ironically losing his capacity for compassion and empathy. He forgot his promise to Shirley and to his family and lost all sense of balance.

"Our worlds grew apart," Shirley went on. It devastated me, and I could see it destroying Roger too, but he denied it, just as our fathers had. When I suggested he get counseling, he snapped. He tuned me out. Everything I said or did annoyed him. I realized I had lost him to medicine, just as I had lost my own father and he had lost his. I was alone, and I would need to do everything on my own or my family too would be destroyed."

"I can see why you're not able to rest." I paused. "Have you feared being alone or had difficulty sleeping before?" I asked.

I've never had problems sleeping, but my fears go back to childhood," she answered and then continued.

My mother spoke about how "she had nothing." It wasn't true, but she believed it, and it consumed her just the same. When my father moved out, she began hoarding anything and everything she could. To this day she saves everything. You can't walk in her home or open a closet door without a collapsing tower of stuff eating you alive. If you offer to clear it out, she acts like you threatened to shoot her first-born. My mother worships her stuff as if doing so will preserve her family. I can't stand the thought of stuff replacing my family, but I would die before I let my family down. I pledged I would prioritize them but didn't think I would be doing it alone. Now I am to become the mother and the father for our children, but I feel too exhausted to be anyone. My body won't move, but my mind won't stop racing. My back pain is flaring, and I'm getting headaches and feeling nauseous every day. I have so much to do I can't rest. I don't have time, and I don't want a divorce.

Shirley's speech gradually slowed, fading like her words. "If I could just rest. . ." She shut her eyes.

My words jolted her, "Let's get you a good night's sleep and talk tomorrow." Her exam was normal, and she denied self-medicating or using any substances. Reluctantly, she agreed to ten milligrams of Ambien and a taxi ride home.

The next day Shirley jogged five miles back to the office to get her car. She confirmed she had slept well and said she felt guilty for having ranted. She assured me she would be fine and was so much better, after just one good night of sleep. She agreed to use the Ambien again if she had another bad night and to follow up the next week.

## Insomnia

Anyone who has suffered from acute or chronic insomnia and experienced the resulting cyclical fear of not sleeping appreciates the value of a good night's sleep. Adequate sleep plays a role in physical and mental well-being and promotes clear thinking and optimal performance. Sleep deprivation poses a major risk for developing cognitive difficulties, excessive daytime drowsiness and accidents, and subsequent chronic health problems, including anxiety, depression, obesity, respiratory disease, and heart disease, if it becomes chronic (lasts more than three months).[159] The Centers for Disease Control and Prevention (CDC) reports that only 65 percent of adults get the minimum recommended seven hours of sleep nightly and over 30 percent of Americans suffer from chronic insomnia. There are many causes of acute and chronic insomnia, including sleep apnea, substance abuse, chronic pain, medications, anxiety, stress, depression, post-traumatic stress disorder, swing shifts at work, and time-zone travel.

In Shirley's case her fear of divorce and losing herself and her family were sources of intense stress and precipitating factors for insomnia. She fitted the criteria for acute insomnia defined by the International Classification of Sleep Disorders: difficulty falling asleep, difficulty staying asleep, or early awakening despite the opportunity for sleep, associated with impaired daytime functioning, that occurs at least three times per week for at least one month but less than three months.[159,160]

Initial treatment often includes taking medication, addressing underlying conditions, and prioritizing good sleep hygiene, which includes exercising regularly (but not within four hours of bedtime); avoiding large meals and fluids in the evenings; limiting caffeine, tobacco, and alcohol four to six hours before bedtime; using the bedroom for sleep and sex only; maintaining a regular sleep-wake cycle of at least seven hours nightly; and avoiding loud and bright stimuli or extreme temperatures at bedtime. For patients with chronic insomnia, a sleep diary, relaxation training, and cognitive behavioral therapy (CBT) can be effective complementary treatments to assist in understanding and overcoming excessive and troubling thoughts that prevent rest. The words of Ralph Waldo Emerson can be used for calmly affirming the time to sleep: "Finish each day, and be done with it. . . . You have done what you could."[161]

By the time Shirley saw me a week later, she was again exhausted.

"How is your sleep?" I asked.

"I don't have time to sleep," she said, pushing her frizzed hair aside and revealing bloodshot eyes. "I have so many things unfinished. I haven't had time to talk to Roger, and now . . ." she paused. "And now he is moving out, and I'm packing his stuff at night, because there is no time in the day."

"Can you describe your average day?" I asked.

I get up at five o'clock every day, without an alarm. I make breakfast, which often no one eats, and I offer to drive the children to school, but they usually walk or take the bus. I leave the house as soon as they do and volunteer at the homeless shelter each morning until eleven. I take calls on the women's shelter hotline most afternoons or meet on board projects if I am not on the hotline. I lead a Girl Scout troop two days a week, after school, even though my daughter has dropped out. I help coach Little League soccer, which my son used to play. I make dinner each night, although, as with breakfast, often no one eats it. At night I work from home. While the children do homework, I make committee calls and write or review reports. Occasionally, I go back out to art shows or meetings of the school board. I try to go to sleep at eleven, but recently it seems useless, so I work at the kitchen table until two or three, or I linger on Facebook or just gaze at the screen.

"Are you exercising?"

"No," she answered.

"Are you at least eating the meals you prepare?"

"Sometimes, but I hate to eat alone."

"Do you get any time with your children or Roger?"

"The children don't want to do anything together, and I can't find time to talk to Roger." She sighed, throwing up her hands.

Shirley's reaction to Roger's shutting down was to do more. Losing the most meaningful aspect of her life resulted in her losing balance. Torn between hopelessness and incapacitation, she coped by overachieving. Her to-do list was now driving her. She was obsessed with fear of losing purpose and was robotically completing tasks to mask her fears and needs. Along her trail of giving, Shirley had lost control of her time and was watching her life unravel, as she feared. Exhaustion limited her judgment; it owned her and, paradoxically, became her wake-up call.

"Would you be willing to devote a little time to completing a sleep diary and time log?" I asked. "The goal is to understand how you spend your time and get back time for what matters to you."

"What does that entail?" Shirley asked.

A sleep diary is simply tracking sleep hours. A 24-7 time log is similar to a food diary, but in this case time and activities are tracked over twenty-four hours for seven days. You list activities by hour in three major categories, with subcategories unique to you. The first category is *S* for "sleep." This starts with the time you commit to going to bed (recognizing for some that might not be the time you fall asleep) and tracks until you get up out of bed. The second is activities done primarily for yourself—labeled as *M* for "me." These activities might include exercise, reading, reflection, eating, or any other purposeful self-time. The last category is *O* for "others" and includes any activities done primarily for others, such as family, friends, community, work, or school. Some activities may overlap among categories, and you decide which category to use. For example, going for a jog with your spouse might be *M* if the main purpose is your own exercise, but it could be *O* if you are doing it primarily to connect with your spouse. Last, you assign a "+" or "–" to each hour of activity to indicate if during that time your tank felt replenished or depleted.

The goal is to track all activities for a full 24-7 period and then review the totals and averages for each day. There is no right or wrong answer, but it is valuable to reflect on how you spend your time and to observe patterns and areas of imbalance when you are overwhelmed. The busier we are, the less likely we are to know how we spend our time, or anything else for that matter. Being busy becomes a cycle, breeding more busyness. Imbalance or a crucible event, such as an impending separation or divorce, becomes an opportunity to assess time, just as you might review your food intake following a change in weight. Saying, "I don't have time" is a red flag indicating you might want to complete a time log.

Shirley agreed to track her sleep and activities hourly for a week and returned the following week with a summary of her log. Shirley used the suggested categories, and she added her own subcategories to include OO for online, OF for family, OC for community, and OD for doctor appointment. She also rated each hour as positive, if she felt it replenished her, or negative, if she felt it depleted her. I was impressed but not surprised with her level of detail. She had given this the same attention she gave to all her activities, and I was eager to reflect on her findings. I asked her basic questions to prompt her learning from this activity.

## Shirley's 24-7 Time Log

"What was your experience in completing the time log?" I asked.

"It took a lot of time," she laughed.

"What went well?"

"I felt good after I slept six hours on Tuesday night, even though on average I slept only four hours a day."

"What else did you observe over the week?"

"I'm not getting much sleep, and I devote a lot of time to others. I also had three doctor's appointments last week, more than I've had in the past year."

"What were your appointments for?" I asked.

"First my back pain flared, so I went to orthopedics, and they recommended ibuprofen, an MRI, and the option to consider surgery. I then went back to the gastroenterologist for worsening nausea. He stopped the ibuprofen, but then my headaches flared up, and so Roger arranged for me to see a neurologist, who recommended a CT scan. But Friday night I slept well and Saturday I went for a run, ate dinner with the family, and felt completely fine. Seemed like all the alarm was a waste of time."

"How is your back and your stomach and headaches now?"

"All fine."

"Good. Were there any other patterns or anything else you noticed?"

"I spend six hours every day on my computer or my phone."

"Did that surprise you?" I asked.

"Yes, and I was shocked to also see how much more time my children spent chained to their devices. They're like slaves."

"Did your hours online replenish you or reflect your priorities?"

"Very little of anything I did last week felt positive or represented what matters to me. I barely had any time with family. I tried to talk to my children, but they were constantly plugged in. I tried to talk to Roger face-to-face about preserving our marriage, but got only texts saying he was so busy. Even when we were all home together, I felt alone. I spent most of my time

SHIRLEY'S 24-7 TIME LOG

| | SUNDAY | MONDAY | TUESDAY | WEDNESDAY | THURSDAY | FRIDAY | SATURDAY | WEEKLY AVERAGE |
|---|---|---|---|---|---|---|---|---|
| TWENTY-FOUR-HOUR TOTALS | 4-S+-- | 2-S++ | 6-S+++++-- | 3-S+++ | 4-S++++ | 5-S++++- | 4-S+++ | 4-S |
| | 6-M+------ | 3-M+++ | 3-M+-- | 4-M++++ | 3-M+++ | 3-M+- | 6-M+----- | 4-M |
| | (6-OO) | (6-OO) | (6-OO) | (6-OO) | (6-OO) | (6-OO) | (6-OO)----- | (6-OO) |
| | ----- | ----- | ----- | ----- | ----- | ----- | (3-OF)+++ | (2-OF) |
| | (2-OF)++ | (1-OF)+ | (2-OF)++ | (2-OF)++ | (1-OF)+ | (3-OF)+++ | (5-OC)----- | (8-OC) |
| | (6-OC) | (11-OC)------ | (7-OC) | (8-OC) | (10-OC)--- | (6-OC) | | (<1-OD) |
| | ----- | ----- | ----- | (1-OD)- | ----- | ----- | | |
| | (1-OD)- | (1-OD)- | | | | (1-OD)- | | |
| DAILY HOURS RECORDED | Pos. 4 | Pos. 6 | Pos. 7 | Pos. 9 | Pos. 8 | Pos. 7 | Pos. 7 | Pos. 7 |
| | Neg. 20 | Neg. 18 | Neg. 17 | Neg. 15 | Neg. 16 | Neg. 17 | Neg. 17 | Neg. 17 |

S = sleep; M = me time; OO = other online; OF = other family; OC = other community; OD = other doctor appointment
"+" = an hourly activity that replenished
"−" = an hourly activity that depleted

doing community projects and rated most of my activities as depleting." She paused. "Looks like I failed this test, huh?"

"Not at all," I responded.

This is not a test. We all get the same 24-7 amount of time, but how we use the time is our choice and varies day to day and week to week, based on our needs and situations. The goal of the log is not to judge how you allocate time but to become conscious of and learn from it. The exercise is a success if you analyze your results and make purposeful change. There are no right answers, but there are some best practices that you can shoot for when you're feeling "out of time." For example, seven hours of sleep daily is recommended for adults, having daily "me" time promotes personal balance, and having a greater percent of activities that replenish rather than deplete is always advantageous.

Shirley nodded.

"What might you do differently to replenish yourself and reallocate your time?" I asked.

"I could increase 'me' time by exercising daily the way I used to, I could try to get us all offline and talking to one another, and I could definitely cut back on some community commitments."

"Excellent! None will be easy, but all three are important to rebalance. Do you know how you will do them?" I asked.

Shirley asked for time to think about her goals and agreed to touch base the next week. I completed a physical exam, which was normal, and congratulated her on her willingness to reassess her time. She thanked me and left. I was still thinking of Shirley when I entered the next patient's room and found a mother and her three young children glued to their devices. Only the mother looked up.

## Technology's Impact on Health

When I look around, everyone is looking down: in meetings, in restaurants, on the streets, in parks, at sporting events, in the library, and even while driving. Being plugged in is the new way of life or, as some suggest, a way of not living life. The American Psychological Association recently linked the "inability to log off" with statistically significant increases in stress over the past decade. Those describing themselves as "constantly checking" email, texts, and social media reported an average stress level of 5.3 out of 10 versus a level of 4.4 for those not constantly linked in. The smartphone, which did not exist prior to 2006, was in 2011 owned by a third of the U.S. population and in 2016 by two-thirds. Nearly half of the population now refers to this device as a necessity they "can't live without." In 2015 the average age to own a smartphone was down to ten, and the average smartphone user spent five hours online and checked her device over one hundred times daily, an equivalent of every six minutes.[162] The World Unplugged Project at the University of Maryland found that the majority of students around the globe experienced increased distress when asked to go without devices for just twenty-four hours, and one in three preferred to give up sex rather than her smartphone.[163]

Connectivity has its benefits, including access to unlimited knowledge and to friends around the globe. Work, thanks to technology, is now often home-based and flexible, but the downside to this convenience is that work can be conducted around the clock. Many with flexible hours lose the ability to unplug and are multitasking twenty-four hours a day, seven days a week, and fifty-two weeks a year, in careers extending well into their seventies.

Constant connectivity negatively affects our physical, social, and mental health. This obsession with technology has been referred to as the iDisorder.[14] The more connected we are, the less active we are and the less time we have for nature and face-to-face relationships. Higher rates of social bullying, suicide among middle school students, and isolation are also linked to constant connectivity, and the CDC reported that over the past decade the rate of suicide in middle school children had doubled and surpassed the rate of death from motor-vehicle accidents.[164] One hypothesis for this rise in suicide is the increase in cyberbullying, which is exponentially worse than real-time bullying because the message—true or not—is heard not just by one or two people but potentially by millions across the Internet community.

Users of social media receive a constant barrage of "Likes." Every day young adults send more than one hundred texts, and thousands of users of blogs, Instagram, Snapchat, and Twitter go online frequently and for great lengths of time to validate their worth. Facebook recently hit a billion users on a single day, and YouTube users upload four hundred hours of videos every minute. Being plugged in provides immediate satisfaction, with a dopamine rush of instant pleasure that drives users to crave more. Whether for pleasure or FOMO (fear of missing out), 87 percent of millennials report their smartphone "never leaves their side."[165,166]

We don't know what the long-term benefits or harms will be, but we know our future will definitely hold more technology, as advanced and easy-to-use products are on the rise. Our challenges going forward will be to (1) be conscious of what we are giving up, knowing that more time online means less time for something or someone else, (2) establish boundaries that allow this tool to complement and not deplete our lives, and (3) know when to turn it off, so that we, like our phones, can recharge as needed.

## My Experience of "Getting to kNOw"

In 2008 I was at a peak in my academic career at Dartmouth. I was serving as section chief, chief clinical officer, and vice chair of my department, director of our regional primary care center, member of the NH Board of Medicine, and medical director of the Office of Community Based Education and Research. I was encouraged to apply for the medical school's leadership scholarship to complete a master's in public health. I fell prey to the culture of FOMO (fear of missing out) and gave my most comfortable response: yes. *The word no* was not in my vocabulary. I ignored the unsolicited feedback of family and friends asking, "How can you do all that?" I was a proud multitasker and viewed those warnings as pessimistic.

But as I began Paul Batalden's systems-improvement course and engaged in the personal-improvement project, I found myself saying, "I don't have any time" for anything—my patients, students, children, and even myself. My health, which I had taken for granted for nearly fifty years, began to show wear. Not diseased but not optimal either, I categorized myself as "at risk." My sleep became disrupted, my diet poor, my previously habitual workouts scanty, my to-do list undone, and my relationships tense. I struggled to create a project goal, for fear of doing more. I began to ask myself, what matters? This was a new concept for me, as I had previously responded yes to all requests without considering time limitations or consequences. I began by generating a priority list, which, more the irony, had "health" as number one: an area in which I was an expert and which I had previously modeled effortlessly but had recently taken for granted.

Dr. Batalden's words to our class, "an invitation is not a mandate," empowered me, and I titled my project "Getting to kNOw." My goal was to explore and improve my process of making choices hour to hour and day to day and to increase the rate at which I said no to nonpriority options. My ultimate aim was to free up time for things that mattered, and my hypothesis was that using the unfamiliar word *no* more often might provide coveted time. I was correct, and I learned in just six weeks that time spent "Getting to kNOw" provided high return on my investment. I discovered that my use of time could determine my health and that, like everyone else, I have only twenty-four hours a day in which to live my life. I can do anything, but that doesn't mean I must do everything, and more multitasking (no matter how good I believed I was at this) would not benefit my family, my patients, my team, or my health.

## Shirley's Experience of "Getting to kNOw"

Shirley returned a week later and reported that her sleep was improving. She had shared her log and goals with her children and Roger and had acknowledged to them that fear was having negative effects on her health. She showed her vulnerability and told them how afraid she was of losing them. Roger always took off the last week of August before school started, and he suggested that the family go away together. They had previously gone to their home on Cape Cod, but he guessed that Shirley would be reluctant to go there, and so he recommended a camping trip. Her children had fond memories of fishing and campfires and agreed. Shirley booked a cabin in Maine and was pleased to be warned by the owner that there were no TVs or Wi-Fi in the rooms. "I am letting you know," he told her, "so your kids will not be surprised." Shirley was thrilled, recalling beachside restaurants on the Cape with tables full of people communicating through devices only. She wanted her family to focus on one another.

In Maine, after a few awkward days reframing their routines, the family rediscovered their bond. Without distractions, Shirley achieved all her goals in one week. She exercised every day: swimming, kayaking, and hiking with her family. They ate three meals a day together and played cards, Monopoly, and backgammon every night. At the end of the week she had caught up on sleep and had a plan to transition out of her role as Girl Scout leader and soccer coach and to cut back on her hours volunteering. She was overjoyed when her son asked to go back to Maine the next year and Roger suggested they not wait until the next year.

She had long walks and talks with Roger and learned that he never expected to be forgiven. He told her he regretted repeating his father's behavior and was shocked that Shirley had not abandoned the family the way his mother had left him and his father. The following week Roger moved back home, saying he had never wanted to leave but had assumed Shirley expected he would. He continued to work, but made it home for dinner many nights and returned to sharing patient cases, engaging the children with stories, and, as they were now older, he added in some surgical gore.

Shirley began "device-free dinners," first on Sundays and then every day. She challenged her children to device-free evening competitions to see who could unplug the longest, awarding prizes of movie tickets and pizza parties to the monthly winners and their friends. She returned to playing tennis and golfing and found that Roger and the children were fierce opponents on the court and on the green.

Three months later Shirley repeated a 24-7 time log and reported hitting a magic number of six. Six hours of sleep, six hours of me time, six hours of family time, and six hours for the community. Her goal, she said, would be seven hours of sleep, six hours of me time, six hours of family time, and the rest community work, some of which she now did with family. Not only was Shirley sleeping better, but she was having less back pain and no headaches or nausea. She was still giving time to others but was feeling replenished in doing so. She was "getting to kNOw" her genuine Super Woman.

# TIME LOG

| TIME | DAY 1 | DAY 2 | DAY 3 | DAY 4 | DAY 5 | DAY 6 | DAY 7 | | |
|------|-------|-------|-------|-------|-------|-------|-------|---|---|
| 0:00 | | | | | | | | | |
| 1:00 | | | | | | | | | |
| 2:00 | | | | | | | | | |
| 3:00 | | | | | | | | | |
| 4:00 | | | | | | | | | |
| 5:00 | | | | | | | | | |
| 6:00 | | | | | | | | | |
| 7:00 | | | | | | | | | |
| 8:00 | | | | | | | | | |
| 9:00 | | | | | | | | | |
| 10:00 | | | | | | | | | |
| 11:00 | | | | | | | | | |
| 12:00 | | | | | | | | | |
| 13:00 | | | | | | | | | |
| 14:00 | | | | | | | | | |
| 15:00 | | | | | | | | | |
| 16:00 | | | | | | | | | |
| 17:00 | | | | | | | | | |
| 18:00 | | | | | | | | | |
| 19:00 | | | | | | | | | |
| 20:00 | | | | | | | | | |
| 21:00 | | | | | | | | | |
| 22:00 | | | | | | | | Weekly totals | Daily averages |
| 23:00 | | | | | | | | | |
| S total | | | | | | | | | |
| M total | | | | | | | | | |
| O total | | | | | | | | | |

S = sleep; M = me time; O = other time; "+" = replenishes; "–" = depletes

## HEALTH CHALLENGE #7    Complete a Time Log

Until you value yourself, you will not value your time.
Until you value your time, you will not do anything with it.
M. SCOTT PECK

The next time you find yourself wishing you had more time, complete a time log to assess your time usage. Track all your activities for one week and then review your weekly totals and daily averages and reflect on the following questions. List activities by hour in three major categories: *S* for sleep, *M* for me, or *O* for others. Create optional subcategories as appropriate to you (OF for family, OO for online, OW for work, OS for school, etc.) Last, assign a "+" or "–" to each hour to indicate if that hour of activity replenished or depleted you.

### 24-7 TIME LOG REFLECTION QUESTIONS

1. What was your experience completing a 24-7 time log?
2. What is working well? What is not working well?
3. What would you like to have done more of?
4. Did you notice any patterns in your day?
5. What did you observe over the week?
6. What surprised you?
7. What did you learn about yourself?
8. Does your distribution of time represent your priorities and values?
9. What might you do differently to reallocate time toward what matters to you?

•  •  •  •  •  •  •  •   •   •   •

# NURTURE A HEALTHY ENVIRONMENT

*Peace comes within the souls of men when they realize their oneness with the universe.*

BLACK ELK

David was heavy for a man in his thirties—not in size, but in mood. He carried the weight of guilt like an albatross around his neck. He described his ache like a shackle pulling on his head, his heart, and his gut. He claimed that it held him more strongly than gravity. It was a chore for David to eat and a chore for him to speak. He had no desires, just heaviness. Once an avid biker, top-notch hiker, and a passionate fisherman, he equated himself when I met him with being the bait, pulled to the bottom of the river by a sinker. He'd been held down for so long he couldn't break free.

David was actually a small man in size—five feet eight and 155 pounds—when he came to my practice. He managed to go to work every day, grateful for the robotic nature of his daily routine. He reported anhedonia, the loss of enjoyment, and he performed only the automatic motions that coincided with living. He described his day as much like a checklist, altered only by being on call every third night.

- Up at five, coffee—black
- Work
- Home at eight
- Read to kids
- Movie with wife
- Bed at eleven

David married his high school sweetheart after college and has two young children. When he came to me for care, he was at the end of his first year of a cardiology fellowship, having completed three years of a pediatric residency, four years of medical school, and four years of college. He had moved to each new program with the hope of returning home to practice after training.

Growing up in rural North Carolina, David had loved to fish and hunt. He had participated in fishing tournaments year-round and had won a local fishing championship at age eleven. At a small college in North Carolina, he began hiking the Blue Ridge and Appalachian Mountains. In medical school he took up biking, and in residency, surrounded by athletes, he biked or ran daily. While in residency, he maintained his outdoor activities with family and colleagues and viewed himself as productive and confident, and a model of health.

But since his three-year fellowship began nine months ago, he had barely seen daylight. He hadn't fished in three seasons, and his habit of cycling or running midday had ceased during the first month of his fellowship. He felt shamed by his peers if he made any efforts toward self-care, as no one in his program took breaks, not even to eat. Guilt aborted all consideration to get outdoors, and he claimed, with a poker-straight face, that his only physical activity was "running behind."

During his time as a fellow, guilt filled every crevice of his day, leaving no space for anything else. He had guilt from not doing enough at work, at home, for his team, or for himself. He feared he was not good enough to be a doctor and called medicine a big disappointment. The slump that he once thought would pass had been going on "forever," leaving him no hope of its ending. He described a dark hole that he had fallen into, where there was no view of the sky and no way out. The life he imagined had been derailed by missed moments that he couldn't recapture. He viewed his life in two parts: eighty-plus hours of work weekly and "everything else." The "everything else" encompassed his unfulfilled dreams: personal integrity, an active lifestyle, strong family time, and a close-knit team. David pointed to the leaves falling outside the window of my office. "Just as leaves wilt and die, so do I," he said. His voice, flat and heavy, showed neither regret nor complaint.

David's program director noticed his performance falling and strongly suggested he see a primary-care provider. David chose me; he had previously attended a wellness workshop I delivered for residents and fellows. David shared that he was struggling to stay awake in conferences, complete his documentation, and engage with patients and colleagues. He acknowledged that he was feeling down and had lost fifteen pounds. In my office David completed a depression-screening survey and answered "absolutely," when I asked Christine Maslach's single screening question: "Do you feel burned out from your work?"[22] I completed a history and physical exam and recommended that he undergo a few basic tests to rule out organic causes for his symptoms.

A week later David's wife joined him for a follow-up appointment. She cried as she spoke. "The man I married is gone, and I can't get him back." His anguish at seeing her distress was palpable, and he attempted to calm her by explaining his feelings, acknowledging, "It's not that someone has died; it just feels that way."

David's labs all came back normal. He knew before I suggested it that his feelings of guilt and anhedonia were classic symptoms of depression. He denied a prior diagnosis but acknowledged a family history of depression, and further questioning revealed numerous episodes in the past decade of hopelessness, irritability, fatigue, and withdrawal from activities. David admitted to feeling so bad that he didn't want to get up in the morning, but he knew where I was going with my questions and adamantly denied suicidal ideation.

## Burnout, Depression, and Suicide in Medicine

Burnout starts early in medical school and continues into all stages of training and across all disciplines of medicine; resident burnout has been reported to be as high as 60 to 75 percent. While no one is immune, some have the skills to overcome it.[17,51] A survey on burnout in physicians and the general working population in the United States between 2011 and 2014 looked at work-life balance. Just as physicians' reported burnout increased to 54.4 percent, while the general public's remained stable at 28 percent, physicians' satisfaction with work-life balance declined to 40.9 percent, while the general public's increased to nearly 60 percent.[17] Burnout exists along a continuum that begins with loss of balance and results in compassion fatigue. It includes hopelessness, physical and emotional exhaustion, depersonalization, dissatisfaction, disengagement, and poor performance and often ends with depression.

Depression is a chronic disease, like diabetes and hypertension. According to the World Health Organization, major depression is one of the most common mental disorders and carries the heaviest burden of disability among mental and behavioral disorders.[167] A full 10 percent of the U.S. population suffers from depression annually, with one in four women and one in ten men experiencing depression in their lifetimes. Estimates are low, as many, including health-care providers, avoid medical care, owing to the stigma associated with the diagnosis. Triggers for depression can be genetic or environmental and include major and chronic stressors. The risk of depression is higher in those with chronic disease, positive family history, or past depression. Having two episodes of major depression leads to a 70 percent chance of experiencing a third, and having three episodes carries a 90 percent chance of having a fourth.[168]

Depressive symptoms vary by individual and were described before their criteria became formalized by medicine. In *Lincoln's Melancholy*, Joshua Wolf Shenk researched Abraham Lincoln's mood, reporting, "No element of Mr. Lincoln's character was so marked, obvious and ingrained as his mysterious and profound melancholy. His melancholy dripped from him as he walked."[169]

Depression can have fatal consequences and is considered the primary risk factor for suicide, with 15 percent of depressed patients committing suicide. Suicide does not discriminate; it is present in all ages, genders, and ethnicities. The CDC reports that rates of suicide are higher for white female physicians, older white male physicians, and all dentists than in the general population. While females have higher rates of suicide attempts, nearly 80 percent of all completed suicides are carried out by males.

A lab partner of mine in medical school jumped from our twentieth-story dormitory. His note said medicine wasn't his calling, and he had to get out. In my residency one resident overdosed and another drove off the highway. Since I have been in practice, I have also lost two colleagues, one found in his garage with the car running and the other in his office with a needle in his arm. All left notes.

Preventing suicide requires recognizing depression. The U.S. Preventive Services Task Force recommends screening all adults and adolescents, in-

cluding all pregnant women at their first prenatal visit.[170] The Patient Health
Questionnaire (PHQ-9) is an easy-to-use, self-administered and scored stan-
dardized tool valid in primary care to assess severity of depression and to
monitor treatment progress. The two-question version (PHQ-2) is more effective for screening than the PHQ-9, with a sensitivity of 97 percent versus 61
percent, but less effective for diagnosis, with a specificity of 67 percent versus
94 percent, respectively. A yes response to either PHQ-2 questions (listed below in the Health Challenge) should prompt additional diagnostic evaluation
with the PHQ-9, which assesses the nine criteria for the diagnosis of major
depression.[171] The PHQ-9 is free and available in over thirty languages. On
the PHQ-9 individuals who score high (above or equal to ten) are between 7
to 13.6 times more likely to be diagnosed with depression by mental-health
professionals, and those scoring low (equal to or less than four) had less than
a one-in-twenty-five chance of having depression.[172]

## DSM-5 Depression Criteria

The PHQ-9 is based on diagnostic criteria for major depression as outlined
by the American Psychiatric Association.[173] Criteria include having at least
five of the following (including the first or second, which reflect the PHQ-2)
for over two weeks:

1. Depressed mood (feeling down, depressed, or hopeless)
2. Loss of enjoyment (anhedonia; little interest or pleasure
   in doing things)
3. Weight or appetite change
4. Sleep changes
5. Psychomotor changes (restlessness or slowing)
6. Poor energy
7. Feelings of guilt
8. Poor concentration
9. Thoughts of death

Strategies for treating recurrent depression often include a commitment
to long-term medication and counseling and, when possible, repeating past

therapies that worked, as they are likely to work again. The pathway out of depression varies by individual, and strategies include assessing the individual's thought processes and interpretation of experiences, coping skills, behaviors, and attitudes, as well as environmental factors, all of which aid in understanding the patient's acute and chronic stressors. Evidence-based strategies to reduce burnout in medical students, residents, and physicians can complement efforts to prevent and treat depression.[25,35,40,53,56,174]

Those suffering with depression may be overwhelmed by the smallest of tasks. In the majority of patients, treatment for six to nine months is necessary and successful. For recurrent or relapsing depression, treatment may be required for at least two years. Treatment is most successful when approached comprehensively and collaboratively by primary-care providers, mental-health counselors, and nurse case managers and includes the use of antidepressant medication and monitoring, psychotherapy, cognitive behavioral therapy, stress reduction, exercise, and close follow-up.[175–177]

On his initial PHQ-9 David scored an eighteen and answered yes to both screening questions. I reassured him, as I do with all patients, that depression is a medical illness, not a character defect or weakness; recovery is the rule, not the exception; and treatments are effective and can be found for nearly all patients. We discussed the complexities of depression and the relationship of stress to physical, emotional, and mental health. We discussed the diagnosis, treatment options, and goals; the duration of treatment; side effects; and recurrence as well as relapse.

David rejected my suggestions to scale his work back to part-time, stating that the option was "unacceptable for men" in medicine. He also declined to take time off, as this would not be tolerated in his program unless the work was done, and the work was never done. He also rejected counseling. The stigma of depression was too great, and, besides, he knew all the local therapists and had no time to go farther away for treatment. With pressure from his wife, he reluctantly agreed to medication and monthly follow-up exams. He was also willing to discuss internal and external factors that he believed contributed to his recurrent symptoms. I described the root-cause analysis process and asked David to consider factors that limited or threatened his wellness. It took him only minutes to create a cause-and-effect fishbone diagram, which listed many triggering factors.

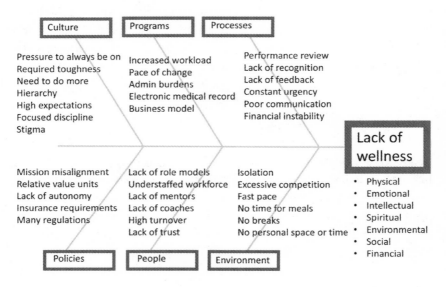

For the past twelve years David had been in intense, competitive, and stressful medical-training environments. David was at the extreme spectrum of burnout and met the criteria for depression. He described his past work environments as demanding and unrealistic at best and destructive and degrading at worst. He attributed hopelessness to the lack of autonomy in his own schedule, unclear expectations around scholarship and publishing, a never-ending clinical workload, and perceived personal inadequacies in teaching. I learned that David had countered previous episodes of feeling heavy by turning to hiking, biking, and fishing. He had previously been rejuvenated and recharged regularly with support from his wife, family, and team, but as a fellow he lacked the time to do anything for himself, his family, or his colleagues.

In his current environment he had lost self-confidence and had become afraid of failing on all fronts: failing his team and patients, failing his family, and failing himself. He'd done nothing for his own health for so long that he could barely remember his priorities. He feared he had let his wife and children down so many times that he couldn't risk doing it again, and he had no faith that anyone on this new team shared his commitment to personal balance. David could more easily see himself disappear than make a change, yet again he denied suicidal feelings.

Familiar with David's achievement-driven culture, I worked with him to set a limited number of attainable goals with the bar low enough to ensure his success. I asked him, "What do you love to do that you wish you were doing now?"

He replied, "Fishing."

"Are you willing to go fishing?" I followed.

"No," he replied.

"Are you willing to get out your fishing gear?"

"No."

"Are you willing to read a fishing magazine?" I said, surprised at his frank honesty and again lowering the expectations.

He paused. "Yes," he offered. He also agreed to take a week of vacation, which he would otherwise lose, as he had not taken any time off yet that year. He set a third goal to find a colleague who he believed modeled personal wellness.

## Treatment Months One and Two: Gone Fishing

We spoke on the phone weekly in the first month after that visit, and David reported compliance with his medication and progress on reading fishing magazines and planning a week off. At the end of the second month, he came in feeling significantly lighter, having succeeded in two of the three goals. His PHQ-9 score was eleven. He and his family had spent the previous week camping on the coast of North Carolina, and he had fished every day with his son.

"What did you catch?" I asked.

"Fishing," he said, "is not about catching the fish but about the experience. It's about being outside and appreciating nature."

"Oh, I see. . . . It was a success even without a fish?" I hesitated, beginning to see a blossom of a personality I had yet to know.

"Actually, I caught six redfish, three bonitos, and eight bluefish." He smiled.

## The Healing Power of the Natural Environment

Environment matters, and the healthiest environment is nature! Biophilia is an innate connection human beings have to other living things. For centuries those connected with nature have reported calmness, positive spirits, pleasure, and reduced stress. But without explicit evidence of its effectiveness, as with nontraditional and pseudoscientific therapies, physicians shy away from prescribing it. Evidence-based literature on the health effects of being out in nature is slowly emerging. Roger S. Ulrich, PhD, a pioneer in using objective testing in research, formed the stress-reduction theory in 1979 that was the basis for numerous fascinating scientific studies that now confirm what has for so long been experienced but not proven.[178,179]

The article "Flourishing in Nature: A Review of the Benefits of Connecting with Nature and Its Application as a Wellbeing Intervention" summarizes current studies that demonstrate the health benefits of contact and interconnection with nature. "Biotherapy," or contact with nature, for even minutes at a time decreases levels of stress hormones such as cortisol, lowers blood pressure and heart rate, increases vitamin D, improves immune functioning, and positively affects energy levels, focus, anxiety, depression, weight loss, diabetes, attention deficit disorder, heart disease, and even cancer.[19]

*Your Brain on Nature*, by Drs. Eva Selhub and Alan Logan, describes details of numerous research studies showing that individuals exposed to natural environments have definite health benefits. That exposure can include brief walks in the park, viewing nature scenes, having access to windows in hospital and prison settings, contact with all types of flora and fauna, and exposure to outdoor activities and more green space over a lifetime. Exposure to nature improves physical and emotional functioning and perceived life satisfaction and lowers physiological levels of stress—as documented by MRI and EEG patterns in the brain, EMG readings of tension in muscles, skin-conduction tests, and blood tests. In addition to the physical and emotional effects, cognitive benefits also come from a deep interconnectedness with the fundamental principles of nature.[180,181] John Muir, known for his belief that nature is essential to well-being, is quoted as saying that "tired, nerve-shaken, over-civilized people could experience awakening while wandering in wilderness."[182]

Accepting our relationship within a larger cycle of life promotes balance, nurtures personal appreciation, and fosters a sense of internal purpose. Many focus on their role in nature to define who they are and their purpose in life. Buckminster Fuller, a Harvard-trained scientist and inventor who popularized the geodesic dome, identified intensely with his role on our planet. After contemplating suicide at age thirty-two, he reexamined his life, in search of the principles governing the universe, and devoted his life to fulfilling the part that only he could play. Day and night, winter and summer, and fall and spring are all examples of balance and rejuvenation that relate to human life. The twenty-four-hour daily cycle, the seven-day weekly cycle, and the twelve-month seasonal cycle provide opportunities for natural renewal with built-in points for balance. With natural balance also comes recognition and acceptance of life and death and gratitude for the time we have on this earth.

Unfortunately, the rates of mental-health problems are skyrocketing, and many who would benefit from nature's therapy have less exposure to the outdoors than ever before. Nature withdrawal and deprivation create vulnerabilities to physical and mental stress, particularly when people live in environments that are not nurturing. Colin Capaldi and colleagues warn of the loss of interconnectivity and express concern about society's movement away from nature. This, they believe, has three causes: urbanization, increased screen time (as we discussed in lesson 7), and destruction of natural environments.[19]

David's vacation, spent fishing and camping, provided him with the benefits of reconnecting with nature. His mood improved, and his love of nature and of family was reinvigorated. His wife and he reconnected and found joy in being together. But his symptom of guilt at work persisted: guilt for not doing more, guilt for not doing less, and guilt for dumping on his team while he was away. David entered his second year of fellowship feeling a bit more confident in his commitment to himself, but he still viewed his work environment as hostile. At the end of his visit, I reiterated the importance of continuing the medication and congratulated David on reconnecting with nature and his family. His progress was beginning to restore his balance and health. I asked David to again focus on his third goal and find a colleague who also valued and modeled personal wellness.

## Treatment Months Three through Six: Hiking, a Win-Win

In David's third month of treatment, we again spoke by phone. His heaviness continued to lift like a morning fog. On the PHQ-9 he scored a seven. As his mood lifted, his family connections strengthened. He was now hiking with his wife and children on the weekends he was not on call, and his successes kept him going through the long workweek. He now understood that caring for himself was good for his family's health.

David reflected on the link between his mood and his environment and began to recognize how his work also affected his health and vice versa. Thoughts of being trapped in the hospital contributed to his feeling of being broken and withdrawn. As is true of many who suffer from depression, David's thought patterns had become distorted. He had overgeneralized ("this always happens"), personalized ("this is my fault"), and magnified with negativity ("this is so unbelievably, horribly bad"). He feared being judged by others for needing or wanting a break. He claimed that his fear sat on him like an ogre, prohibiting him from feeling welcome or engaging. He believed that everyone else was balanced, and only he lacked "integrity" and was unable to achieve health at the level he demanded of his patients. The word *integrity* in Latin means "whole." As integers are whole, we too can be whole when we have integrity. Being "in integrity" in the context of health refers to balance. Maintaining wholeness is difficult in harsh environments, as we lose focus, ignore what matters, disengage, don't contribute, and feel guilty, only to repeat the cycle until balance is lost.

Environment is a physical setting that comes with a cultural expectation of how to act in that location. In David's experience, when in the woods, people observe and reflect, and when in the hospital, people ignore sensations and work robotically. David loved being a doctor and felt stuck. Working outdoors was not an option but neither, he realized, was working every day in his current setting. "How do you stay healthy without feeling guilty?" he asked me.

"Sometimes, I don't," was my short answer. "But if I tell myself that it is irresponsible to *not* model health for my team, my students, and my patients, I often succeed. You could say I shame myself into making time for me. On busy days I still have guilt over exercising, but my guilt is a driver and incentive for a win-win. Being rejuvenated, I thrive in a positive cycle, which makes me more effective in supporting others. I also try very hard to publicly congratulate others who model healthy behaviors: take time for lunch, breaks, walks, and even vacations. My small gestures of recognition seem to go far, as colleagues let down their guard, drop their 'I'm fine' responses, and acknowledge genuine needs. I then feel proud instead of guilty for my own healthy behaviors."

David said, "I'm overwhelmed by the mask of denial worn by my colleagues. I see their immunity to illness as a lie and their omnipotence as a deterrent to reaching out."

"I agree. But I also believe we are our culture, and our culture is us—nothing more! We must empower one another to remove our masks, recreate our environment, and change the scenery."

"So you think I can take care of me despite the predominant culture of neglect?"

"Absolutely! Your taking care of yourself can even change the culture. Modeling is contagious, and leaders who model are also permissive. I totally believe in the power of one. Have you tried sharing your successes with people at work?" I asked him.

"No," David confessed, his eyes turned down. But I saw a glimmer of hope. David admitted he had wanted to share his experiences with colleagues but hadn't had the courage. He compared his current work environment to previous settings and admitted all were stressful, but this one was particularly difficult, as no one talked about personal needs. It seemed an unwritten rule not to verbalize struggles. In talks with his mentor, topics were limited to performance review and career plans, never broaching feelings or fears. For all he knew, he was the only one overwhelmed.

One Thursday afternoon, as his team was rushing to a morbidity-and-mortality conference, the chief resident, Craig, asked David about his recent vacation. David's defenses immediately went up, but as they walked Craig expressed an interest in fishing and not in David's absence from work. David shared a bit of his experience, and to his surprise the chief communicated his own passion for hiking and his struggle to find personal time. Craig walked out of the conference with David and mentioned how he and other residents frequently walked the trails after rounds to survive the long days in the hospital.

In his fourth month under my care, David reported that he had finally achieved this third goal. Craig was his sought-after role model. Hearing Craig's challenges and successes had validated his own feelings and transformed his view of work. David heard from Craig that it was okay to need help, okay to take breaks, okay to go outside in the middle of the workday. David's PHQ-9 score fell to two. Craig's story and friendship gave David the permission necessary to break with the culture and not feel guilty. Craig invited David to join a small group of fellows who hiked regularly on the trails behind the hospital. David was pleased to find colleagues who valued self-care but disappointed to know they wouldn't come out of the closet. David accepted and referred to this group as his "underground" team.

## Environment Matters, Whether Good or Bad, Natural or Built

The health-care environment and culture is saturated with double standards. We preach self-care for patients, but we often ignore the needs of our teammates and ourselves. Learners repeat what faculty leaders do, not what they say. The "no pain, no gain" mentality permeates our culture and stigmatizes anyone who might ask for help that could burden already overburdened colleagues. Health professionals will endure almost anything to avoid being labeled as weak or incapable. *Burden* is a relative term in health systems, as every team member is saturated and cushions are nonexistent; therefore, increasing the workload can only become unbearable. Historically, changes to the system occur only when linked to patient outcomes.

Since the 1984 death of Libby Zion, an eighteen-year-old Vermont college student, medical-residency programs in New York, and nationally starting in 2003, have mandated restricting resident work hours to a maximum of eighty per week and twenty-four continuously and have required attending physicians to be in hospital 24-7.[183] Her cause of death was publicized as a drug interaction at the hands of overworked and exhausted residents. The Libby Zion Law is about preventing error and promoting patient safety. This mandate, while not designed for physicians' benefit, was believed by many to move work conditions in medicine in a healthy direction. Controversy and tension exist between supporters who believe that eighty hours is still excessive if the idea is to guarantee personal balance and opposing factions who believe that limiting hours prohibits effective medical education. Those who are opposed claim that mandating when residents leave the hospital prohibits the continuity and ownership of patients through the evolution of their disease processes and sends learners the message that they can't handle stress. They argue that a resident who admits a patient with chest pain at three in the afternoon and signs off at eight at night will never fully experience the evolution of a myocardial infarction. A 2017 review looking for evidence of the effects of these policies on patients or providers came up short; the ruling was maintained with increased flexibility.[184]

My own family medicine residency at the Medical University of South Carolina in 1990 exemplified a healthy environment. Our program had a required wellness month for third-year residents, who served as backup for residents who needed time off, while simultaneously rejuvenating themselves. The wellness month provided a buffer when a resident needed time away, took a vacation, or even quit (all of which happen in stressed systems). This model allowed individuals to celebrate life events such as having a child or getting married with less guilt and fear of resentment. Unfortunately, this type of program remains rare and is often viewed by other programs as "coddling."

Leaders who value wellness create healthy environments that empower health in all individuals. I was invited to speak at the Family Medicine Department in Denver on strategies to prevent burnout. The topic was fully supported by the chair, who encouraged faculty to take two hours off in the middle of their day to attend and to focus on themselves. He himself publicly blocked daily "me" time on his schedule to reflect and to exercise. The participants, including clinicians, educators, basic scientists, and psychologists, interacted in a way I had not previously experienced. The culture of health created by the chair permitted transparency and support and allowed a sharing of struggles and successes to permeate their overall culture and surroundings. I believe that defining the competency of leadership among health professionals must include the ability to sustain and model personal health.

## Treatment Months Seven through Twelve: Leading Culture Change

Over the next six months David discovered that his "underground team" was constantly and privately struggling to carve out personal time. A faculty member, who admitted to being a closet gym goer, joined their team and acknowledged hiding to avoid bearing resentment. David and I agreed it was better to be judged by others than to become ill for lack of self-integrity. We were both thrilled to see the effects that culture change was having on him and vice versa (even if hidden). He dared to hope that the team would go viral, but the naysayers feared being viewed as slackers.

Knowing that others had similar struggles inspired David to address resistance. He started with small wins, just as he had done personally; he shared his own story and designed a system of cross-coverage (much like a call system) that offered participants one hour of personal time each workday. All could opt in if they agreed to cover one another's pagers. He also initiated a brief personal "check-in," which residents would do as they signed in and out, parallel to the process of rounding on patients. They began to hold one another accountable for *not* being available when they weren't on call, frowned upon doing work at night or on weekends, and strictly forbid the use of work email or pagers on vacations. It didn't take long before word of their successes spread. Their stress decreased as their commitment to one another increased. David also sensed an increase in communication around patients, as they were cross-covering more often.

By his third and final year of fellowship, David had gained back not just his love of nature but also his love of work and his empathy for others. To be a doctor, one must be a leader. To be a leader in health, one must sustain and model wellness. By being true to his love of fishing and hiking, he changed his own health and inspired others. He discontinued his medication, enjoyed time with his family, and scheduled his last follow-up appointment. David's environment felt different to him, and he reported feeling like a model of health himself. He learned to recharge while at work and to totally refresh on weekends and during time away. His guilt diminished, and he perceived his workload as doable.

David's greatest success in changing the culture came when his program director asked him to revise the traditional performance-review process to include criteria for commitment to personal health. David suggested recognizing individuals for taking daily breaks and regular vacations. He also detailed a point system for those who supported health in others and suggested to the director that he and I deliver a monthly workshop on strategies for self-care.

A healthy environment promotes personal balance and prevents burnout. Healthy individuals create a healthy environment. Expanding evidence-based strategies for modeling self-care is integral to sustaining well-being among health professionals, our families, and the patients to whom we are accountable. The downstream impact will be dramatic, with potential for effects on rates of depression, alcoholism, divorce, and suicide for all who are part of the culture.

I believe, based on my own and David's journey to sustained health across settings, that we create our culture. While environment is a physical place, it is also a collection of our thoughts and behaviors. When I think of David now, I see a leader: one who no longer fears his environment and who changed his culture. He achieved balance in his life and modeled healthy behaviors, and as a result improved his own health and the health of those around him. I am grateful to David for validating the importance of my own modeling. I trust that, together, he and I and many others will transform the culture of medicine to ensure health for all.

•  •  •  •  •  •  •  •  •  •  •

HEALTH CHALLENGE #8    Model Wellness

*Men seek seclusion in the wilderness, by the seashore, or in the mountains— but nowhere can man find a quieter or more untroubled retreat than in his own soul; above all, he who possesses resources in himself, which he need only contemplate to secure immediate ease of mind—the ease that is but another word for a well-ordered spirit. Avail yourself often, then, of this retirement, and so continually renew yourself.*
MARCUS AURELIUS

Begin this challenge by assessing your risk of burnout and depression. Ask yourself the single burnout question and the two screening questions for depression. Then reflect on your environment, and consider your connection with nature and the culture of wellness in your working, playing, and living situations. As you complete this exercise, note any areas for self-improvement and contemplate steps that you can take personally to maximize a healthy environment for you, your family, and your colleagues.

# CAUSE-AND-EFFECT FISHBONE ANALYSIS OF THREATS TO WELLNESS

*What individual factors threaten wellness?*

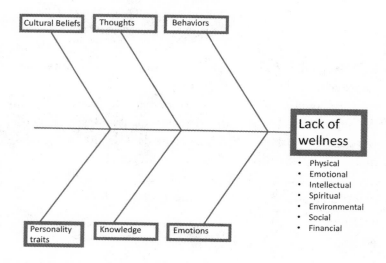

*What systemic factors threaten wellness?*

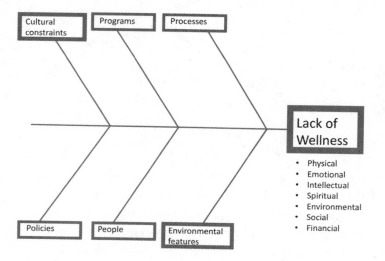

1. "Do you feel burned out from your work?"
2. Over the past two weeks,
   a. Have you felt down, depressed, or hopeless?
   b. Have you felt little interest or pleasure in doing things?

(If you answered yes to any of these, set up an appointment with a primary-care or mental-health–care provider for further screening and evaluation.)

Reflect on your interconnectedness with nature to enhance your natural environment:

1. How can you spend time closer to plants or windows in your home? In your workspace?
2. When is the best time every day for you to go outside?
3. What can you do outdoors on your next day or week off?

Understand the culture of your personal and professional environments:

1. Whom do you observe each day who is a model of health?
2. Complete an environmental SWOT. What strengths, weaknesses, opportunities, and threats to wellness exist in your home, play, and work environments?
3. Complete a cause-and-effect fishbone analysis. Identify internal and external factors that limit your physical, emotional, intellectual, spiritual, environmental, social, or financial dimensions of health.
   - What personal cultural beliefs, thoughts, behaviors, personality traits, knowledge, or emotions contribute to these limitations?
   - What systems-level cultural constraints, programs, processes, policies, people, or physical environmental features contribute to these same limitations on health and wellness?

# PART THREE  SELF-IMPROVEMENT

• • • • ▶ • • • ◕ •

*We can change the world simply by changing ourselves.*

JON KABAT-ZINN

Self-improvement is purposeful change that occurs when we acknowledge a personal gap and take action to better ourselves. The self-improvement process begins with setting concrete personal goals and includes authentic decision making, prioritization of healthy choices, flexibility in thinking, and monitoring of progress and obstacles; it concludes with sustainable transformation and celebration.

● ● ● ● ● ● ● ● ● ● ●

# EMBRACE CHANGE

To exist is to change, to change is to mature, to mature
is to go on creating oneself endlessly.
HENRI BERGSON

George was a seventy-year-old retired gentleman who came to see me for a persistent cough. He was tall and fit, with thinning gray hair and dark piercing eyes. His shirt was carefully pressed, his shoes recently polished, and his tie perfectly knotted. George had gone most of his life without seeing a physician—that is, from a patient's viewpoint. He saw physicians daily, as he himself had been a practicing oncologist until three months before seeing me.

I knew George professionally and over the years had cared for numerous patients that he had referred to me for primary care. Five years prior to his first visit, when his insurance mandated it, he listed me as his primary-care physician, but he had never been in to see me. Everyone called him "Dr. George," not out of familiarity but out of inability to pronounce his Greek last name. Dr. George was one of the few remaining old-time physicians in our hospital. His reputation among his peers was that of a great diagnostician who valued traditional medicine, a knowledgeable academician who worked from his brain (not a device), and a direct communicator who told patients exactly what to do. The millennial generation saw him through a new lens, viewed him as patriarchal, and silently labeled his style on rounds as doctor-focused, not patient-centered. They disagreed with his teaching that "doctors are to be tough and that they need to tell patients what to do."

In my office Dr. George was now the patient. But when he arrived, he corrected my assistant on the pronunciation of his name and gave his title as "Dr. G." He refused to see my medical student and sat at the desk in my chair.

I forgave him for appropriating my seat but was taken back that he refused my student an opportunity to learn. Teaching physicians' unwritten rule is to remember that we too were once students and to make every moment a teaching moment. Even my own experience with labor and delivery of my children was no exception.

George greeted me with his agenda: "I just need an antibiotic and a chest X-ray." He gave me a "you could be my daughter look" and leaned back in my chair. He made it clear that my diagnostic input wouldn't be needed, just my access to the system, as he could no longer place orders himself.

"Nice to see you," I greeted him and persisted with my usual questions, hoping he would respond.

He reluctantly described four weeks of congestion, sore throat, and head-aches, all of which had begun to resolve but had flared again last week into a productive cough, fever, and fatigue. He denied any shortness of breath, rash, or travel. He acknowledged having zero energy and a ten-pound weight loss, which he adamantly attributed to eating healthier since retirement. His past medical history was negative, aside from an appendectomy in his twenties: no asthma, no heart disease, and no allergies. His family history was unremarkable: no cancers, and everyone lived into his nineties. George was divorced, remarried, and currently fully retired. He had pseudo-retired five years ago but had continued to work a few hours every day until three months ago. When asked, he acknowledged that he had two daughters, whom he had not seen in a decade, and a son in California, who often attempted to connect, but whom Dr. George had visited only once, when his first grandson was born. He hastily denied having any plans for his retirement, muttering that he might take a trip, as he had missed his second grandson's birth. Dr. George lived with his second wife, Stacy, who was eighteen years his junior and still worked as a nurse manager. I convinced him to submit to an exam-ination, which revealed a faint expiratory wheeze and coarse crackles at the left lower base of his lungs; all else was normal.

With the exception of his weight loss, which I could accept as consis-tent with a major change in eating habits, his symptoms were classic for community-acquired pneumonia. Eager to meet his requests, I confirmed that he took no medication and had no allergies, before ordering albuterol and a course of antibiotics. Skimming his scant medical record, I paused only to reread a past note for "tobacco cessation." An electronic error, I thought to myself. Half paying attention and embarrassed to be asking, I made a note to correct the record later, while I stated the obvious. "You're not a smoker, are you?" I criticized myself for asking a leading question, while also wondering why I was even asking this of my senior colleague—who happened to be an oncologist.

"Occasionally," he responded, capturing my full attention, bringing me back to high-alert doctor mode.

"What would be an average day?" I asked calmly, red flags going up all around me.

"A few cigarettes now and then," he said, piercing me with his eyes but circumventing my question.

"How many today?" I pushed.

"Two," he admitted. It was nine in the morning.

"Have you tried to quit?" I continued.

"A few times, not successfully. I know the blah, blah, blah—no need to cover that. I'm seventy, and no point in quitting now."

What was he thinking? Did he really believe he was immune? His smoking was beyond my comprehension, and now he was my patient. One of the most powerful lessons I have learned is I cannot force change on anyone. Change must come from within, and my role is limited to that of coach. "Would there be any benefit to quitting? Any advantages you could see?" I queried.

"No, I've smoked for years, and oddly enough, this is the first time I've been sick. I probably should go back to work." He paused, then said impatiently, "I just need an antibiotic."

I feared the worst, but accepted his no for now. I resolved that, if nothing else, a bad outcome would at least strengthen my argument to quit. We agreed on a chest X-ray, a course of antibiotics, an inhaler, and, at my insistence, a follow-up appointment in one week. I assured him of the obvious: "The fewer cigarettes the better." As he left, my thoughts again cycled. Did he not see red flags—a smoker with a cough and weight loss? Did he not assume and fear the worst, as I had? Would his X-ray confirm pneumonia or reveal a large mass with disseminated metastases? Would we spend his next visit exploring reasons to quit and how he would spend his retirement, or discussing which oncologist he preferred to see?

For twenty-four hours my fear persisted, and I hovered over his medical record, awaiting results. Despite my vigilance, he got the report before I did and he sent me a note: "I saw the X-ray and feel much better. I look forward to seeing you next week." Why was he coming back, given that his results were normal and he was improving? Was he feeling relief from fear or just from his symptoms? Did he not believe he had beaten the odds, and did he want to quit? Was he expecting me to pound the facts, give him a quit date, and dictate a plan for him?

## The Why and the How of Change

The process of change is complex and not often amenable to a quick fix. Although we may wish to change others, we can directly transform only ourselves. Change is a two-stage process; first is the why, and second is the how. Identifying a why is often the limiting stage, and, without clear purpose, action rarely occurs, results are variable, and rates of noncompliance are high. For those ready and eager, the how is simply a process of mastering specific and concrete steps. Failure to recognize a patient's stage of readiness often results in futile efforts.

The following week Dr. George arrived on time, my last patient of the day. His shirt was pressed and shoes shined, but the tie was missing. He stood as I entered and reached out for my hand, his piercing eyes softer. "Thanks for seeing me," he said and sat in his chair. I sat in my chair by the desk.

"I'm glad you're back. How are you?" I asked.

"My cough is better, I've had no fevers, and I'm not nearly so exhausted," he reported.

"That's great. You look good. I was relieved to see the pneumonia. I worried it would be worse and should order a CT scan to screen for lung cancer," I added.

"My weight is up two pounds. I'm going back to the gym shortly. There was nothing suspicious, right?" he asked.

"Nothing." I reassured him. "But you're high-risk, and the guidelines are for all men and women ages fifty-five to eighty who have smoked on average a pack a day for at least thirty years and are current smokers or who have quit within the past fifteen years to have an annual low-dose lung scan."

"Okay," he agreed.

"I'm impressed you get to the gym. Is that new?" I asked.

"No, but I go more since I've retired."

"Congratulations on making time to exercise. Does your wife go with you?"

"Occasionally."

"What else do you enjoy doing together?" I asked.

He smirked. "We both smoke."

"Have you ever talked about quitting together?" I prodded.

"I know what you are going to say, so save your breath," he said. I sat in the chair opposite him, feeling a wedge between us. Stung by his direct style, I took a deep breath before speaking again. I would push him. "You know there is value in me, as your doctor, explicitly advising you to quit.[185] So I have to say it. Quitting smoking is the number-one thing you can do to improve your health—you must quit smoking!"

"Thanks, I know!" He nodded and coughed.

Did he resent my telling him what he already knew? George, the doctor, was cognizant of the harms of tobacco. Since the 1960s the U.S. surgeon general warning has been on every pack of cigarettes, making the harmful effects public knowledge. Most people who smoke do so despite knowing the danger, and even despite experiencing the ill effects of cigarettes. Most also underestimate the magnitude of potential harm to themselves. The CDC reports tobacco as the leading cause of death in the United States, accounting for over 430,000 deaths annually (or one in every five). Tobacco use also results in a reduction in life expectancy of 5.5 minutes per cigarette smoked (five to eight years lost on average).

Dr. George also knew that subsequent surgeons general have reported that quitting smoking has health benefits across a lifetime, no matter what age you quit, even after age sixty-five. Improvements in lung function and reduction of cough and congestion occur within as few as three months after quitting. By the one-year mark, a former smoker's risk of vascular disease is reduced by 50 percent, and after fifteen years it is exactly the same as a nonsmoker's. The risk of lung cancer and other forms of cancer are reduced by 50 percent just ten years after a smoker quits.

"Fifty years ago," he continued, "when I was in college, everyone smoked, and it relaxed me. I cut back when I had children and my first wife hounded me, but I picked it up again when she left. I smoke more when I am alone. When the hospital went smoke-free, I hoped that the policy would have a greater impact, but it served only to send me into hiding. I stopped socializing and went home frustrated. I smoked in the morning and at night and used nicotine gum at work."

"What do you like about smoking now?" I asked.

"It makes me less irritable—I could use one now!" he snapped.

"What makes you irritable?" I nudged gently.

"The usual stress," he said. "Life, work, family."

"Has the stress decreased since you retired?" I asked.

"No, it's worse," he replied.

"Worse?" I repeated.

"I have nothing to do and no purpose. I'm agitated all the time and I smoke more."

"Sounds as if you don't like being controlled by cigarettes but don't have other priorities to keep you busy. Is there something else that could replace cigarettes in your life?" I reflected.

"I don't know! You're the doctor," he snapped again.

To be honest, the cigarettes are all I have left; everything else is gone. Cigarettes are my one consistency and distraction in life, and sometimes they feel like a companion. When my first wife left years ago, she took the children with her; I dived into my work and I smoked—not much else. I was never much of a father; my kids don't exactly admire me. I'm not much of a husband either. My current wife, Stacy, intended to retire with me, but we don't do well at home together. I'm pretty irritable, so she went back to work, and I wouldn't be surprised if she left, too. The only thing I was ever good at was being a doctor, and that's gone. So there's my life, and I'm not really interested in having you force me to give up "my cigarettes."

"I appreciate your sharing, and I'm not going to force you to do anything," I said, mirroring what I heard. I wasn't certain I had the skills in my black bag to motivate Dr. G., but I decided I would try my motivational style and give him, as the patient, the control. "If I understand what you are saying, you have mixed feelings about smoking. Your career has been a success, but you have lost your family's respect and connections, and since retiring you have also lost your sense of purpose. Cigarettes have been your mechanism for coping with the stress of loss and are a source of comfort. On the other hand, while you know tobacco is unhealthy, you exercise regularly. You also don't like the idea of anything or anyone controlling you, but you fear that you are dependent. Is this accurate?" I asked.

"Very."

"If you had other options, you might choose not to smoke?" I suggested.

"I might."

I was beginning to understand Dr. George's ambivalence. His thoughts, feelings, and physical needs were intertwined, blurring his decisions, but it was clear he needed to lead his change.

## Motivating Someone to Change: The Why

Understanding what motivates people is fundamental to fostering change. Fear is a great motivator, but we are not motivated by fear alone. As Daniel Pink, author of *Drive*, describes, the drive to change is linked to an individual's (1) autonomy: desire to control personal decisions, (2) relationships: commitment to those they value and love, (3) mastery: aspiration to be an expert in an area, and (4) meaning: quest to live purposefully.[186] Motivational interviewing (MI), as defined by William R. Miller and Stephen Rollnick, is a "skillful clinical style for eliciting from patients their own motivation for making changes in the interest of their health." Their 2013 book, *Motivational Interviewing: Preparing People for Change*, is considered the MI bible.[187] MI is both an interviewing style and a practical set of counseling skills shown to assist coaches in helping others recognize unhealthy behaviors and adopt new ones. Linking new behaviors to personal desires, commitments, aspirations, and sense of purpose enhances the victory. MI is effective across a variety of conditions and is applicable in all aspects of life.

The MI approach, originally introduced by the psychologists James Prochaska and Carlo DiClemente, is built on three principles: autonomy, guidance, and alliance.[188] The task of the physicians or coaches is to guide patients to identify what it is they want to change, to clarify a personal reason to change, and to support them in making the change. A strong interpersonal alliance between the physicians and patients is fundamental to success; this collaboration relies heavily on an empathic style of communication and active listening.

In this model, ambivalence is recognized as normal. Using MI techniques, a coach assesses the pros and cons of a given behavior by asking open-ended questions and fully listening to the patient's response. Overcoming any indecisiveness is achieved by tipping the scale toward a positive behavior aligned with what motivates the patient: autonomy, relationships, mastery, and purpose. The MI model suggests that what motivates one person is not necessarily what will motivate another. This principle makes understanding each patient's thoughts and fears, as well as passions and values, critically important. It is vital to remember that behaviors are driven by feelings, not just by thoughts, and that ambivalence is not limited to cognitive processes. At the core of all emotion is the voice of human need. Internal conflicts driven by fear must be understood in order for change to take place.

"What do you fear?" I asked Dr. George.

"Nothing."

"What keeps you up at night?" I asked.

"It bothers me that I don't have enough time to repair the damage I've done to my family. My son is just like me—I know he is struggling, but he won't ask for help, and, given my own gaps, I don't know that I have much to offer."

"Who says you don't have enough time? Why not go see him?" I asked, adding, "You said you needed a purpose."

## The Emotional Component of Change

The nonsmoker relies solely on intellect and makes the claim, based on facts, "I would never smoke." But for even the most educated smoker, a personal decision to quit is not so simple; the smoker must overcome the battle between an internal voice of reason and that of feelings. Emotional arguments to smoke often conflict with intellectual arguments to quit. Rational thinking is undermined by stress. Feelings can be more potent than beliefs, and fear often trumps fact.

It is human nature to elude pain and seek pleasure. Habits like smoking are used to mask unpleasant feelings and deep-seated fears, like the fear of failure, weight gain, inability to cope, depression, anxiety, loneliness, chaos, abuse, and death. Facing intense emotions is arduous, particularly when one's training emphasizes thinking over feeling. Although life presents a plethora of experiential learning opportunities to practice coping with intense feelings, our culture in general and the field of medicine specifically undermine these learning opportunities with not-so-subtle messages: be strong; ignore your emotions; hide your weaknesses; limit vulnerability; don't feel sad, tired, hopeless, hungry, overwhelmed, or even happy—just keep *doing* more and you won't *feel* anything.

Emotional intelligence (EI), coined and described in 1990 by Peter Salovey and John Mayer of Yale University, is defined as a "form of social intelligence that involves the ability to monitor one's own and others' feelings and emotions and to use this information to guide one's thinking and actions."[189] Their model includes four abilities:

1. To identify and express both one's own and others' emotional states;
2. To understand and analyze emotions;
3. To harness emotions to facilitate their use in all situations; and
4. To manage emotions both in oneself and in others.

Daniel Goleman, author of *Emotional Intelligence: Why It Can Matter More Than* IQ (2005) and coauthor, along with Richard Boyatzis and Annie McKee, of *Primal Leadership: Unleashing the Power of Emotional Intelligence* (2013), is considered by many to have started the movement to know one's feelings, suggesting that EI was a critical leadership skill.[190,191] Leaders in health care, however, often learn to intellectualize their fears and develop a sense of invincibility, further distancing themselves from emotions. Too much knowledge can also give a false sense of immunity from disease and permission to ignore medical guidelines. The neurosurgeon Paul Kalanithi highlights in his 2016 memoir, *When Breath Becomes Air*, how a physician's knowledge can mask emotions and how emotions can mask knowledge. When Paul first feared he had lung cancer, he intellectualized using data and reassured himself that his risk as a thirty-six-year-old nonsmoker was only 0.0012 percent. When Paul's fears became reality and the diagnosis of lung cancer was confirmed, his emotions flooded him, and gone was his knowledge. He wrote, "Death, so familiar to me in my work, was now paying me a personal visit. Here we were, finally face-to-face, and yet nothing about it seemed recognizable. Standing at the crossroads where I should have been able to see and follow the footprints of the countless patients I had treated over the years, I saw instead only a blank, a harsh, vacant, gleaming white desert, as if a sandstorm had erased all traces of familiarity."[192] EI training includes self-awareness and self-management, with a focus on addressing one's emotions and recognizing the effect they have on one's own behavior and on that of others. It also includes social awareness and relationship management to demonstrate empathy and build strong relationships.

Lacking EI, many mask uncomfortable feelings with excessive anything: work or alcohol, drugs or sex, food or exercise, television or movies, texting or video games, money or gambling, and even compensatory emotions and behaviors, such as anger or violence. Anything in excess that is continued despite causing more harm than good is an addiction. Addictions mask many feelings and fears: drugs mask pain; drinks mask abuse; food masks insecurities; work masks grief; caffeine masks fatigue; exercise masks compulsion; use of social media masks social anxiety; violence masks dysfunction. Certain addictions, such as tobacco, are detrimental to health from the first use, produce dependence with continued use, and result in physiological withdrawal when stopped. The most immediate remedy to eliminate these unpleasant physical symptoms is to reuse.

It was after six in the evening, and my office had closed long ago, but to my surprise Dr. George was still engaged. I wondered, What was most important in George's life and what would tip the scale for him? What purpose could he find? I asked this most basic question: "What and who matter to you?"

"My reputation as a doctor," he replied, without hesitation. "And my health and children," he added. "I don't want to be a doctor who dies alone. But it's too late. I probably have cancer somewhere and my children don't care."

I caught the slightest glimpse of a smile as he pulled a picture out of his wallet. It was a school photo of a young boy—big smile, missing front teeth, bowl haircut, stiff white shirt, and a navy tie. "What is his name?" I asked.

"George, my grandson." His smile broadened.

"How's George?" I asked.

"I haven't seen him since he was born, and I've never met his brother, Alex. My son seems resistant to my neglect and continues to send photos and invite me to visit regularly, but I've been too busy working. I guess I don't have an excuse anymore."

"I guess not," I mirrored.

Our marathon visit ended. Dr. George agreed to think about quitting and to follow up with me. When he returned three weeks later, he declared he was ready to quit and would to do so in the next six weeks. He had called his son, received an invitation to California, and wanted to quit before seeing his grandsons.

## Making the Change: The "How"

I grew up in a goal-oriented family in Camden, New Jersey, and was taught that action mattered. My great-grandparents were from Europe and sought to be part of the American culture. They passed down their commitment to contribute in meaningful and measurable ways to their children and grand-children. My mother, now retired, was a researcher and statistician at the N.J. Department of Health, Education, and Senior Services, as well as a Girl Scout leader and a special-education teacher. My father, a first-generation college graduate, joined the navy and became a lawyer. He spent fifteen years in the U.S. House of Representatives before serving as governor of New Jersey and still teaches and works full-time at the age of eighty. Their combined message to me echoes the words of Eleanor Roosevelt: "You must do the thing you think you can not do!"[193]

MY EXPERIENCE EMBRACING CHANGE AND COACHING PERSONAL HEALTH IMPROVEMENT  Teaching personal health improvement is the most re-warding work I have had in my career as a family physician and professor at Dartmouth College for two reasons. First, my own health and wellness is critical to my effectiveness and performance as a mother, clinician, teacher, and person, and I am personally challenged to continually "walk the walk." Second, I have seen the effect the training has had on thousands of learners—undergraduate and medical students; residents and faculty; and nurses and other health professionals, including nutritionists, psychologists, care coor-dinators, social workers, and health administrators—all audiences universally appreciating the time, the tools, and the permission to focus on themselves.

Having experienced the value of maintaining personal learning plans, I developed a personal health–improvement tool (PHIT). The www.myphit. org website allows individuals to track their projects, sustain their efforts, collaborate with others, and maximize success. Participants around the globe have completed the PHIT plan and are actively working on SMART (specific, measurable, achievable, relevant, and timely) goals. The top ten PHIT themes have surprisingly been similar across audiences, independent of background, age, culture, level of experience, or even training. They include, from most to least frequent:

1. Begin meditation or mindfulness
2. Enhance physical exercise
3. Advance healthy eating
4. Improve sleep hygiene
5. Foster reflection and journaling
6. Unplug from technology
7. Improve time management
8. Increase social supports
9. Promote positivity and appreciative inquiry
10. Start a new/old hobby (read, write, paint, sing)

DR. GEORGE EMBRACES CHANGE    Dr. George was motivated and skilled, and he knew the improvement process well. He was willing to adapt the model he had used for improving systems in the hospital to construct a plan for his own health. His global goal was to quit smoking. He knew what had and had not worked for him in the past, and his SMART goal was to cut out one cigarette every other day for forty days, beginning that day. He mapped the factors that contributed to his smoking to anticipate barriers to his quitting. He identified two metrics to assess his success. The first was a process metric, looking at the action of cutting down. It was a yes-no measure of his ability to stick to his limit each day. His second was an outcome metric, looking at the consequences that mattered. He chose a daily self-rating of irritability on a scale of 1–5 (1 = not at all; 5 = irritable all day). His activities included calculating and purchasing the total allotted number of cigarettes for the full forty days. He would count and place each day's allotted number in a small tin each morning and carry it with him. After the forty days he would celebrate being a nonsmoker. He identified his wife, Stacy, as a resource *he had* and his son, who he believed would support him if he asked, as a resource *he needed*. He left that day with a concrete plan, committed to embracing change. I let him know I was cheering for him and was available if he struggled. I expected George to fully succeed.

Not only did George succeed at quitting smoking, but he also went to California and bonded with his son and grandsons. Feeling confident with his son's acceptance, he reached out and reconnected with his two daughters. He traveled back and forth for a year and then moved to California. His wife continued working in New Hampshire for another year, where I saw her regularly, and she was planning to move to California also. She shared that Dr. George was not surprised to have been diagnosed with throat cancer, but, despite his diagnosis, his quitting smoking had triggered a series of positive changes; their relationship was stronger than ever before, he was a fabulous grandfather, and he was living with one of his daughters. She also shared that he was receiving treatment on the West Coast and had a good prognosis, but that when his time came, Dr. George would have no regrets and would die a happy man, surrounded by his family.

• ● ● ► • ● • • ● ● ●

HEALTH CHALLENGE #9    Initiate a Personal Health-Improvement Tool

To know what has to be done, then do it, comprises
the whole philosophy of practical life.
SIR WILLIAM OSLER

When there is something in your life you believe needs improving, make a SMART change and implement a personal health–improvement project. You can identify a health gap by analyzing your SWOT from lesson 2 and your personal resilience assessment from lesson 3. To optimize your success, visit www.myphit.org to design your plan, track your progress, and receive daily reminders.

1. Global goal: write a broad statement that describes what you want to overcome, achieve, or change.
2. SMART goal: create an aim that is specific, measurable, achievable, and relevant, and that can take place within a reasonable time frame.
3. Likelihood of success: answer the following motivational questions to assess your likelihood of success.
   a. How important is it for you to achieve your goal? (1 = not at all important; 10 = extremely important)
   b. How confident are you that you can achieve your goal? (1 = not at all confident; 10 = extremely confident)

If you rated either question as a 6 or below, consider choosing a different goal.

4. Process map: create a cause-effect fishbone diagram (similar to the one in lesson 8) of the factors that contribute to your current health gap.
5. Measures: How will you know that you've reached your goal? What will you measure and how will you measure it?
   a. Process metric (to confirm that an action has been completed). For example, check "yes" or "no."
   b. Outcome metric (to know if you've made a difference). For example, determine a numerical rating of stress or positivity.
6. Activities to accomplish the goal: What next steps will you take? Will you, for example, purchase a journal or join a gym?
7. Resources to help accomplish your goal: Who and what do you have or need to achieve your goal?
   a. Resources I have: _____
   b. Resources I need: _____
8. Timeline: When can you start, assess, and finish the process? Ideally, start today and go for a minimum of twenty-one days.
   a. Start date: _____
   b. Assessment date: _____
   c. Finish date: _____

*Source:* Adapted from © Center for Continuing Education in the Health Sciences and the Office of Community-Based Education and Research at Dartmouth.

• • • • • • • • • • • ·

# MAKE HEALTHY AND AUTHENTIC CHOICES

*The chief happiness for a man is to be what he is.*
ERASMUS

Lena was a fourth-year medical student who emailed me after attending a workshop I led on sustaining personal wellness across the continuum of medicine.

Dear Dr. Pipas,

Thank you for a great session. I was so grateful to you for sharing your experiences. I walked into class feeling stressed and tired but left feeling rejuvenated and more optimistic! You hit the nail on the head in mentioning what none of our professors yet have acknowledged: "Medical school is draining. Keep at it, you're almost there." I have felt a palpable slump both for myself and among my classmates, and by addressing it up front this morning, you have made it easier for those feelings to be acknowledged, accepted, and—hopefully—uplifted.

I wish I had completed a personal SWOT and vision statement earlier in my training. I have been going through the motions of being a medical student, but never feeling I was doing it right, never in the moment, never enjoying anything, even my pastime of running has felt like a chore the past four years. I am graduating in three months and am so unsure of my future.

I heard about your self-directed wellness elective from a classmate and need a recharge before considering residency. I would love to work with you and look forward to hearing from you.

With gratitude,
Lena Patel, MSIV, Geisel School of Medicine at Dartmouth

Lena requested that I mentor her for a monthlong elective. She committed to reflecting on her medical school experience, weekly readings, and discussions. She had a partial list of readings from past students and wanted help to finalize her list. Lena looked the part of a doctor when she arrived a week later to discuss the elective. She walked confidently into my office, wearing a dark suit, with her long black hair pulled back. I tried to imagine what specialty this striking young doctor would choose.

Her professional confidence evaporated, however, as she began speaking about her experiences in medical school. She wasn't sure she could be a doctor or even that she wanted to be. She wasn't sure she enjoyed anything in medicine or anything at all. She couldn't picture herself as a physician and feared committing to a life sentence of imbalance. Residency match day was approaching, but she would not be celebrating with her classmates, as she had decided to defer.

Lena left my office that day to begin reflecting on her first year of medical school and to read *The Pocket Thich Nhất Hạnh*.[81] At that point all I knew of Lena was that for nearly eight years, she had lived alone in the United States, having left northern India to attend Princeton and then medical school at Dartmouth. Her father, mother, and two younger siblings remained in India, but they visited every July for a month and stayed in her apartment. They would be making the trip this year in June for graduation. Her father had wanted to be a doctor but was instead a successful researcher. He adored Lena and wanted to give her every opportunity he hadn't had. He coached her to "do anything," which Lena interpreted as a mandate to "do everything." Lena often felt torn trying to meet his expectations.

## First Year of Medical School: Overwhelming Expectations

Lena arrived for our first official meeting with notes from her readings on her iPad, ready to share her learnings about her first year of medical school.

SETBACKS   "First year was unbelievably hard. I hadn't imagined the workload," she began.

> Every day I told myself, "I can't do this." I studied until I thought I would go crazy, but I barely kept up. It was like learning multiple foreign languages simultaneously and being immersed in them to drown—alone. I wanted to be the perfect student I had been in college, but I couldn't possibly know everything needed to pass the boards and care for patients, let alone teach or have my own research. Everyone talked about the "imposter" syndrome, but I believed only I wasn't smart enough and didn't belong. I felt guilty for wanting a break and watched myself slip into old habits. My only thoughts were of worthlessness and failing. I skipped meals, lost weight, and feared breaking my promise.

Lena felt that medicine was swallowing her. She recalled her first winter semester as the lowest point of her training. By the dark days of February in New Hampshire, she had lost ten pounds and prayed for a break from the monotony of her classroom and library existence. She longed to exercise but believed that time off could mean the difference between passing and failing.

I shared with her the intensity of my own first year of medical school. I remembered how dark the February days felt in Philadelphia. I had been overwhelmed and disappointed that it was not what I thought I had signed up for: my life consisted of days in the classroom and nights in the library, with not a patient in sight and no life outside of the two-block radius of my school. I had been frustrated that I had no autonomy in my schedule, and I had been angry and resentful of medicine for taking away my life and limiting my ability to participate in my family's lives, only ten miles across the river in New Jersey. I was drowning in medical information, and I remembered distrusting myself, wondering how I had been led down a path so far from what I had imagined doctoring to be.

"How did you survive?" Lena asked.

"I struggled, like you and most classmates. I was frustrated. Midyear, I remember accepting a grade of 'pass' as good and coming to terms with life outside medical school being null. I lowered my expectations, and I told myself daily that I had one priority—learning. I wish I had known then that medicine would be as rewarding as it was demanding. It has brought me great joy and satisfaction but, at times, has left me empty."

"Empty is how I feel even now in fourth year: inadequate, anxious, exhausted, hopeless, and empty," Lena echoed.

"Many in medicine have those feelings. In your class of nearly one hundred students, fifty will feel like you and disengage as a result of burnout. Thirty will become clinically depressed and drop out of the workforce for some time. One will feel so bad he or she won't want to live and will contemplate or commit suicide." I shared with Lena, as I had with David during his residency (see lesson 8), my experiences losing colleagues to suicide as early as medical school and throughout my career.

"Why doesn't anyone talk about this?" Lena asked. "I thought I was the only one overwhelmed. I've worked so hard to get here. I know what unhealthy feels like, and I don't want to go there again. I thought being a doctor would ensure health."

Lena was not unique. The drive for perfection combined with the stigmatization of self-care and of mental-health care are what prevent open discussions on burnout in medicine.

BURNOUT AND EATING DISORDERS   In high school Lena was expected to excel at everything. Her father encouraged her to stand out, insisting that she go to an international boarding school. "Never do anything halfway" was his advice. In field hockey she stood out as the fastest and was invited to join the running team. At first Lena enjoyed running, but as the pressure to win and to get into college increased, running became her world: she ran to relax, ran to stay thin, ran to eat more, ran to be recognized, ran to win, and ran until she no longer menstruated. Depriving herself of food also became a reward: her coach congratulated her on dropping weight, and she was faster when lighter. She aspired to have no body fat and fell from 120 pounds to 100. She viewed fasting as a form of strength and skipped meals. She ignored her body's signals and acquired a distorted "supermodel/superhero" self-image. No one intervened; she was a winner.

It wasn't until she returned home after her senior year of high school that her family's shock caused her to look in the mirror. Her local doctor admitted her and announced she was malnourished, beyond what he saw in the poorest of children. Lena suffered from the athletic triad—disordered eating, amenorrhea, and decreased bone density—that is seen in many female athletes, and she met the criteria for anorexia.[194] Her father forbade her to run; her mother blamed the school's cooking and fed her steadily. Lena blamed herself and feared starting college in the fall. At home that summer she saw a counselor, learned about eating disorders, and gained back ten pounds. She taught English to her siblings and worked as an assistant to her father's research team. She felt strong and made a personal promise to stay that way.

In college Lena avoided team sports, moderated her exercise, ate healthy foods, and returned to 120 pounds. She sought counseling after observing her own past patterns in her friends, who ate no carbs, were "allergic" to all food, competed to exercise more and eat less, drank excessively and threw up, and threw out dishes of food. Lena focused on her image of herself as a scholar and, surprisingly, kept her promise. Learning about eating disorders and watching her classmates suffer led her down the premed track.

Like many medical students, Lena came to medical school at the top of her game physically, emotionally, and intellectually. She had excelled at Princeton and was determined to do the same at Dartmouth. But the desire to be perfect led Lena to exhaustion by the end of her first year. While she craved recognition for her hard work, all she could see were her shortfalls. Familiar patterns of asserting control in the face of overwhelming demands resurfaced, but with no time to run, all she could control was her food and her weight.

"Did you go for help?" I asked.

"No, I was too tired to care and chose medical school over me. I broke my promise to myself."

Unrealistic expectations, vulnerability to loss of control, and personal inadequacy are common in both burnout and eating disorders. Both populations are susceptible to unrealistic expectations (a desire to know it all or to be a size 00), barraged by irrational self-criticism and flagellation at not achieving the unachievable (perfect grades or the body of a supermodel), and prone to depersonalization, with denial of feelings, including compassion for self and others ("I'm not tired or hungry" or "He doesn't need help"). Both are therefore at risk for disengagement and isolation to protect their "secret failures" (too busy studying to socialize, too tired to run or to eat, not worthy of support or acceptance) and susceptible to physical and emotional exhaustion, poor performance, and an increased risk of depression and suicide. Burnout results from a "chronic mismatch between people's perceptions of workload, control, rewards, community, fairness and values"; these perceptions can be more potent than actual work conditions in negatively affecting work-life satisfaction.[18]

The etiology of eating disorders includes genetic, cultural, environmental, and stress-related causes often linked to unrealistic body image and the idealization of thinness. Eating disorders are defined by abnormal eating habits that negatively affect a person's physical or mental health. They occur ten times more often in women than men, with up to 4 percent of girls experiencing bulimia or anorexia over a lifetime. Onset is often in the teens, and symptoms occur in nearly 10 percent of college females.

Two of the most common and serious eating disorders are bulimia nervosa and anorexia nervosa. Bulimia is characterized by binge eating, purging, and excessively evaluating self-worth in terms of body shape or weight. Anorexia is characterized by lack of maintenance of a healthy body weight, an obsessive fear of gaining weight or a refusal to do so, and an unrealistic perception or nonrecognition of the seriousness of low body weight. Severe anorexia can cause menstruation to stop, but this is not a requirement for diagnosis.

The SCOFF five-question tool, described here, can be used by clinicians to screen for eating disorders.[195] Two or more affirmatives to any of the five questions warrant further clinical evaluation.

1. Do you make yourself Sick because you feel uncomfortably full?
2. Do you worry you have lost Control over how much you eat?
3. Have you recently lost more than One stone (fourteen pounds) in a three-month period?
4. Do you believe yourself to be Fat when others say you are too thin?
5. Would you say that Food dominates your life?

Lena faced increased risk of burnout and disordered eating. She watched helplessly as symptoms surfaced. She feared gaining weight even when underweight and feared failing herself and her family, even while succeeding in an Ivy League medical school. In our initial meeting Lena acknowledged an overwhelming fear of never being happy. She thanked me for listening and for sharing and left my office committed to finding peace and to reflecting on her second year of medical school.

## Second Year of Medical School: Alone

Lena returned the following week, having read *Drive: The Surprising Truth about What Motivates Us*, by Daniel Pink.[186] Reflecting on her second year, Lena said that she had developed a rhythm of studying and her grades were fine, but she recalled that there had been nothing else in her life. She had lost more weight and reported feeling disengaged and, paradoxically, bored.

"Did you have friends in medical school?" I asked.

"No," she answered. "Everyone was supercompetitive, supersmart, or superstudious. The supercompetitive always had to have one up on one another, more time in the lab, less sleep, better grades. They were always gunning for the dean's list and entrenched in competing. The supersmart were laid back and seemed to do it all; they excelled academically, socially, and athletically. The superstudious studied nonstop. I was none of those. I didn't belong." She paused.

"Besides, I was forbidden to date. I hoped for a nontraditional 'love marriage,' but my father refused and was arranging my marriage. While I was here, he would consider family background, education, financial status, and land, among other factors, and choose my mate. Unlike my cousins, I lacked the 'right of refusal.' My husband would be announced in my absence." She shared that she could "do anything" except question her father's decisions.

I had not realized the complexity of Lena's family traditions or the depth of her cultural ties. Reflecting on her isolation, I recalled how much support I had required from friends in my second year. Classmates who were also struggling were eager to bond and study in groups. We laughed at ourselves during late nights in the library trying to learn the Krebs cycle, only to forget it again, joking that it was unlikely to save anyone's life. After exams, which

I still painfully remember as being scheduled every Monday, we always took a night off and went out in Philly. We reminded one another how lucky we were to be at Jefferson Medical College and how important our future work would be. I don't know that I would have made it through without my friends.

"Did you have support in second year?" I asked.

"I called home weekly," Lena responded. "But at school I thought I was the only one feeling that way until I saw my classmates' anonymous postings on our Facebook page. They talked about taking time off, and one classmate wrote, 'Not even my best friend knows I am on antidepressants.' I gave all I had to the looming boards and passed, but there was literally nothing left to me; my weight was an all-time low of 98 pounds."

No one noticed Lena fading away. She was alone and made no call for help at a time when supports were vital. Lena requested and was granted a year off. Her grades were strong, so it was a simple application. She chose not to go home but to spend a month at a silent retreat in Barre, Massachusetts, then to work at a research lab in Boston. Her father agreed only after she emphasized that the research would increase her chances for a top residency slot. She provided the excuse of living with a roommate to deter her family from visiting that summer.

After deciding to defer her third year, Lena realized how important personal choice was as a driver of success and happiness. Following her father's rules had been ingrained in her since birth, but Lena felt she had little choice regarding her career, her future marriage, or the direction her life was going. She couldn't question her father, and she criticized herself for not succeeding. She needed to recharge. She left my office, still thinking of second year and still wondering what choice she had now, at the end of her fourth year.

## The Year Off: Building Resilience

Lena returned a week later, having reflected on her year off from medical school and having read Drs. Steven Southwick and Dennis Charney's book, *Resilience: The Science of Mastering Life's Greatest Challenges.*[7] She shared: "I learned a lot about myself that year—I realized how much I loved research and time for me. I tried to imagine what I would do if given the choice to stay or leave medicine." During that year Lena contemplated not returning to medicine but feared being rejected and ostracized from both the medical and the Indian culture. Failing was as unacceptable for her as requesting a divorce, which in her culture occurs in only 1 percent of marriages versus 45 percent of those in the United States.

That year was the first time she had seen a photo or learned about Raj. She had received a letter from her father announcing her marriage. Raj was handsome and four years older than she, upper middle class and from her hometown. He was completing a PhD in India at the same research center as her father. She could not refuse, and thus no response was expected or given from Lena. This was fait accompli. Family and friends received the announcement in person, as her father arranged for it to be delivered at every door in the neighborhood. In her third year Raj was invited to join her family on their next visit to the United States to meet her. Lena recalled having mixed feelings as she read of her father's joy and her future marriage. "I knew my family would choose well for me, but I felt trapped between cultures—blessed to be Indian and in America, but cursed not to fit in or have a say in my future. I was excited and horrified."

Reading *Resilience*, Lena also realized that acceptance and positivity were strengths of hers. She knew she couldn't change her father's decision, and she accepted his arranging her marriage. His effort on her behalf was a gift and protected her from the pressures of dating and the ticking of the fertility clock felt by classmates. She trusted her family, and so she focused on her career decision. Looking back, Lena realized how happy she was during that year off. She had read about the "paradox of choice" and agreed that even with food choices, having "too many" options did not increase her happiness.

Lena recalled that when her gap year ended, she felt recharged and eager to return to her third year of medical school, which she heard was clinical and much more like being a real doctor than the first two years. She was thrilled she was going to be with patients and out of the classroom. She was looking forward to choosing a career specialty that included research and to finding a balanced mentor. She left my office that day ready to reflect on her third year of medical school, feeling excited about her future and again promising to maintain balance.

## Third Year of Medical School: Searching for a Role Model

Lena returned a week later, having read *Wherever You Go, There You Are*, by Jon Kabat-Zinn.[59] The long-awaited third year had not been a relief for Lena, but another disappointment. What she found beyond the library walls scared her into wishing she was doing research again. "I entered the clinics and was shocked at the culture of self-neglect and self-abuse all around me—students bragging about not sleeping, residents competing for who had more meals from a vending machine, and senior faculty who were mostly divorced or working part-time. 'Welcome to the war zone' was my greeting to medicine wards. It seemed unreal that in the medical culture everyone had to be a rock to survive. My supervising residents were cynical, with one announcing the first day of surgery that his goal was to weed out those of us who couldn't cut it."

Her search for a role model also came up empty. The doctors she worked with were robotic, going nonstop from dawn to dark. They complained about administrative pressure and referred to the good life before electronic records. They claimed it was impossible to adequately care for patients. To her, they seemed imprisoned and to prefer that everyone around them was also miserable. She was surprised when attendings labeled classmates as lazy and shamed them for prioritizing themselves above medicine.

"Why," Lena asked, "if doctors are the health experts, do so many burn out?" She knew the literature and had seen firsthand that burnout was not due to lack of knowledge or skills but to an acceptance of culture, practices, and attitudes. We spoke of the desire to fit in. Medicine, Lena observed, was powerful, prestigious, and seductive, and it was eating her colleagues alive.

Lena shared her sadness at how little appreciation anyone received. All she heard was "You're not working hard enough." Everyone talked about enjoying life, but appeared frantic and overwhelmed. Medical professionals were held in great esteem and looked on as superheroes, but she did not want to fill superhero shoes; she wanted a specialty that rewarded her for being herself. Lena's ambivalence about perfection and balance superseded her happiness in her work. She was also introverted and found each clerkship block with a new team exhausting. By the middle of her third year, she was again worn out. "Are any specialties immune from burnout?" she asked.

"None are immune." I answered, wondering if my answer would relieve or add to her fears. Burnout does vary by specialty, but it is present in 50 percent on average and increased across all specialties between 2011 and 2014. The highest rates are seen in emergency medicine, urology, and rehabilitation, with family medicine ranked fourth. The lowest rates are in radiation oncology, pediatrics, and psychiatry.[17]

"Should I go part-time?" Lena asked. "Is that the only way for me to be a balanced doctor?"

"Going part-time is one option. Students, residents, and faculty may choose this for many reasons, including to decrease stress and provide a balance at times in their lives—I have chosen this myself," I acknowledged. But I also shared that going part-time could add stress and would not be enough to bring joy to work that was not fulfilling.[196] Lena's questions brought back a flood of memories.

As a resident, I had lived alone and managed my workload. I hadn't minded long days, nights on call, or weekends in the hospital because I found joy in my team and my patients. I had been focused and was doing what I loved. But after residency I married a physician, and two years later, at thirty-two, I had my first child and found myself torn between work and family. When I was pregnant, I considered going part-time and sought advice. My academic mentor advised that I stay full-time for at least six months after maternity leave "to prove I was reliable." Then, if I "couldn't handle the load," he said I could go part-time. A senior colleague, who worked "full-time plus," shared that she was planning to go part-time; her marriage had ended, and she was needed to support her teenage children. Another mentor and full professor advised that to succeed in academia I should hire an au pair (as she had done), so that I could be available around the clock for my department chair and dean. She said, "Do everything requested of you to earn your credentials as soon as possible." My mother's advice was the only instruction to the contrary. She said, "Every day your children are alive, they need you less." The clash of "mother knows best" versus "doctor knows best" forever rings in my ears.

Like Lena, I tried to do everything. I went part-time, but like other part-time colleagues, I worked full-time hours. I tried to be available at all times for everyone. Part-time status bought flexibility on paper and a decrease in salary but often increased stress. I felt inadequate as a mother and a doctor, needing to be home when I was at work, and at work when I was home. But there was still no time for me. I found balance only when I began to make choices that took into account my own health. I gave up obstetric care when my second daughter was born, so that I could sleep and be home at night for my children. When my youngest began preschool, instead of returning full-time, I made the choice to remain at 80 percent. It was one of the most important decisions in my career. With time to focus on me, I found greater purpose as a mother and as a doctor. There was still a cost, but the benefits far outweighed them.

## Fourth Year of Medical School: The Power of Choice

In the final week of her elective, Lena read *The Happiness Hypothesis: Finding Modern Truth in Ancient Wisdom*, by Jonathan Haidt, and she came early to my clinic, hoping to see if family medicine might fit her.[63] I congratulated Lena for performing at the level of a resident, but I saw that she was worn out and showed no joy in her work.

Lena reflected on her current fourth year:

I finally caught my breath but had increasing doubts about my future. I met Raj the summer after third year and spent time getting to know him, and he me. He believed in me even more than I believed in myself and was excited for our future. When my family left, I went to the AAMC Careers in Medicine resource hoping to find the right specialty and guide my choice of electives.[197] But after child psychiatry, emergency medicine, pathology, radiology, and radiation oncology, I was more convinced I didn't fit. I was scared to death when I heard the rumor that going from the fourth year of medical school to internship is like driving your brand new Maserati into a brick wall. I am afraid internship would destroy me and that I'd never succeed with the added responsibility of a family. I've come so far and my father has invested so much money, but I can't see myself here, nor can I disgrace him. Maybe medicine is not for me.

She read a 2017 article I recommended titled "Association between Physician Burnout and Identification with Medicine as a Calling." The author concluded, "Physicians who do not identify with medicine as a calling experience more burnout."[196] Physicians were surveyed to understand the association of a "sense of purpose or calling" in medicine with the likelihood of burnout. Compared with physicians who reported no burnout symptoms, those who were completely burned out had lower odds of finding their work rewarding, seeing their work as one of the most important things in their lives, thinking their work makes the world a better place, enjoying talking about their work to others, choosing their work life again, and continuing with their current work even if they were no longer paid (if financially stable).

Choosing the right career is critical to your health. An authentic career match increases a sense of purpose, productivity, work-life balance, and happiness. In studies on burnout in nurses, job satisfaction had an inverse correlation with emotional exhaustion and the desire to leave health care.[24] The importance of job satisfaction is increasing, given the alarming rates and costs of stress-related disability, job turnover, absenteeism, and presenteeism in America. Many believe that the key to this decision is doing what you love and loving what you do. The American author and journalist Paul Krassner shared, "One of the aspects of happiness is when you can make as little distinction as possible between your work and your play."[198]

When Lena asked, "Should I be a doctor?" I was surprised at the simplicity of her question, and I thought of the complex decision made by students, residents, and colleagues I have known who have left medicine. I thought of how many choices we make every day without formal consideration. Career decisions are major choices and warrant reflection and an intentional method to examine potential gains and losses. Making the right choice matters, as the right choice promotes health, builds relationships, and enhances happiness and productivity.

Lena and I spoke about the many facets of her decision. A traditional method of making choices is based on importance and urgency. This model works well from a perspective of increasing productivity and running a business. Employers may prefer this model if a job needs to be done immediately. An alternative model of making choices is based on wellness and authenticity. Decisions based on this model are made by asking yourself two questions: (1) Does this decision enhance my wellness, or am I well enough to take on this choice (is my tank full)? and (2) Is this decision in alignment with my passion, strengths, and purpose? This is not to suggest that you never do things that are important or urgent, but that in making major decisions like career choices, you look inward and consider your own wellness and authenticity as key in the analysis. "Every decision," I told Lena, "comes with a cost."

## Cost-Benefit Analysis

I urged Lena to explore what she loved, what she was good at, and what provided her with meaning in her life and to assess the costs and benefits of remaining in medicine. Lena's list follows.

Lena spent much of her time in medical school overwhelmed and isolated and without support; she felt she didn't belong. Despite this, she succeeded academically and completed the criteria to receive her MD degree. But it came at a cost; she doubted herself and was increasingly vulnerable. He passion was not as a doctor, and failed attempts to find a role model and a specialty with which she could connect left her questioning medicine as an authentic or healthy career.

Lena graduated from medical school the month after completing her elective with me. After graduation Lena left medicine. She returned to India to marry Raj. She put herself and her health above medicine and hoped her husband and family would support her. Her father was overjoyed that she was a doctor and welcomed her home. She discovered what mattered to her and how best she could contribute to her own health and to the health and wellness of others with whom she would work and live in the future.

### LENA'S COST-BENEFIT ANALYSIS

| Costs of being a doctor | Benefits of being a doctor |
| --- | --- |
| Personal balance | Having family members' approval |
| Short-term physical health (eating disorder) | Prestige with external recognition |
| Long-term emotional health (burnout) | Accomplishment and success |
| Isolation and inability to pursue anything else | Financial independence |
| Continual fear of failure | |

The following fall I received a beautiful note and wedding photos of Lena in dozens of colorful saris.

Dear Dr. Pipas,

Thank you for your support. Raj and I got married and are planning for our own home. I am teaching biology and English. I applied for a research position and am excited that someday my work will impact medicine. Medicine will always have a place in my heart, but I don't miss it. I know I can do anything, but I also realize that I don't need to. I am enjoying my mother's cooking and rereading my elective notes. I know that I will be successful and balanced, because I trust myself. As you suggested, now that I have made my decision, I am focusing only on the benefits. Thank you for teaching me to make healthy and authentic choices.

I miss you!
Lena

My image of Lena will forever be that of a gorgeous bride in a colorful sari. I was disappointed that she did not remain in medicine but overjoyed that she made a personal choice and put her health first. Lena confirmed for me that quests for perfection can undermine health and personal happiness and that making healthy choices is more powerful than doing everything, independent of one's culture. Career choices based on that which you love, that which you are good at, and that which gives your life meaning affect not only job satisfaction but also long-term health and life.

• • • • • • • • • • ⋅

HEALTH CHALLENGE #10  Construct a Cost-Benefit Analysis

The greatest wealth is health.
VIRGIL

Reflect on a choice you currently face and consider the following questions to ensure you make the most authentic and healthiest choice.

|  |  |
|---|---|
| *That which you love* | *That which you're good at* |
| HEALTHY AUTHENTIC CHOICE | |
| *That which gives your life meaning* | *That which provides greater benefit than cost* |

1. What do you love? What are you passionate about? What do you enjoy doing? Is choosing this option likely to make you happy and bring you joy?

2. What are you good at? What are your unique selling points—your strengths, knowledge, skills, styles, attitudes, and capabilities? Refer back to and expand your SWOT from lesson 2. Is this option likely something that you would excel at?

3. What gives you meaning? What would you do even if not being paid, assuming you were financially wealthy. Would doing this give you purpose and align with your values and commitments?

4. What is the cost to you? What will you lose if you make this decision—physically, emotionally, intellectually, spiritually, socially, or financially? Consider short- and long-term effects. How well are you? Are your basics covered—clean water, healthy food, safe environment? Is your tank full and your plate empty enough to take something else on? Is this something you might choose to do but can't do now? Could you do this at another time, when your health is optimal? What is the cost to those who matter to you? What do others stand to lose?

5. What are the benefits to you? What will you gain if you make this decision—physically, emotionally, intellectually, spiritually, socially, or financially? Is there anything to gain by not taking this option? What are the benefits to those who matter to you? What do others stand to gain based on your choice? How important or urgent is it that *you* do this? Are you the only or the best person to do this job? Can you nominate another person who might be better suited?

• , • • • • • • • ◦

# REWRITE YOUR STORY

*People are disturbed not by events, but by the views which they take of them.*
EPICTETUS

Jeff was a twenty-three-year-old college senior who came to me for a physical. I'd known him for many years and had previously cared for his mother, father, and older brother, Scott. Jeff had been healthy and remarkably resilient despite adverse childhood experiences and his father's addiction. "How are you?" I asked.

"Not so well. I failed two exams, and my girlfriend found me passed out and is threatening to break up."

"Passed out?" I asked.

"Yes, from drinking."

I was shocked, recalling how Jeff previously swore he would never touch alcohol. I knew Jeff primarily through knowing his dad, Ray, who was an alcoholic. Ray had tried but failed at sobriety numerous times. When Ray drank, he said things he later apologized for. He told Jeff and Scott they were useless; "good for nothing—like cat piss" were his exact words. He told them, "If you have no money or liquor, you're a loser." Ray had a near-fatal drunk-driving accident roughly four times a year and numerous other odd accidents regularly. He suffered from alcohol-related physical and mental-health illnesses, but despite these outcomes he maintained a mentality that he could have "just a few." For him "a few" meant five or six "hard drinks," as he never counted his daily dozen or so beers.

Jeff recalled how out of control home had felt and how hard he and his mother had tried to make things normal. He had been embarrassed to have friends to his house, and his mother had been devastated at all the relationships his father destroyed. Despite his dad's abuse, the family celebrated every time he succeeded at being sober for just a day. They were convinced they could help their dad, but repeatedly the boys lost faith. Their hope was shattered when he remained sober for only one hour after leaving alcohol rehab centers, or when the next morning they found him passed out on the floor, again. Jeff empathized with his dad, having heard stories of Ray's childhood horrors. He believed his dad's behavior was not excusable but also not incomprehensible given his dad's experiences.

Ray drank to treat underlying anxiety, depression, and low self-esteem. Ray boasted he could cure anything with alcohol: bad day at work, bad day unemployed, bad fight with his wife, bad tension headache. He was known for his saying "I'm drinking my way to being okay." Ray was an only child by the age of six, having lost his older brother in a boating accident and his younger sister to an unknown illness. Ray's parents both drank to ease their pain; alcohol was their cure for the loss of their children, the guilt at having no jobs, their anger for hurting each other, their fear of another DWI, and their general disappointment in life. Alcohol dulled Ray's parents' emotions, including any positive feelings, which were short-lived. Ray was never taught to understand his thoughts or feelings or how to cope with stress. He was never loved or taken care of. His primary lesson as a child was that booze was more valuable to his parents than he was. Ray recalled a calm only at dinner, which he ate alone, while his parents slept between afternoon and evening drinks. Every experience Ray remembered he categorized as "before, during, or after" his parents' bouts of drinking.

Ray's father, Laurence, committed suicide before Jeff was born. Ray's grandmother had previously died of cancer. Ray told the story of Laurence's death every time his sons committed him to alcohol rehab. To prevent them from helping him, Ray threatened to end his life the way Laurence had. Laurence's story, according to Ray, is as follows: Laurence's only wish was to "drink himself to death." He tried again and again and again and again but failed many times. Ray finally stopped caring—it was too painful. Laurence's only regrets were about surviving and being brought to the hospital. He hated the tubes doctors inserted to resuscitate him. He believed the tubes were his punishment for having failed. On his last attempt, he did his usual: drank and then drank more. Only that time, he left a note: "NO

MORE TUBES," crayoned on the back of a Chinese menu. To ensure this, he superglued his mouth and nose shut. By the time doctors intubated Laurence, he was not dead as he had hoped, but he was no longer alive. He "existed" in a nursing home and died a year later.

Ray was barely twenty when Laurence got his wish. At the time, Ray was married to Jeff's mother, and they were expecting Jeff's older brother, Scott. Jeff's mother worked hard to support her grieving husband. She finished graduate school and raised the children like a single parent, because Ray's grief never ended, nor did his drinking. Compassionate and educated, Jeff's mother made every resource available to her husband—the most expensive rehabs, therapists, and psychologists—but Ray believed that therapists were useless. He blamed the world for his problems and was adamant that he could not be helped. He had little hope of sobriety, much less a healthy lifestyle. In spite of their dad's lack of belief in therapy, Jeff and Scott were encouraged by their mother to get counseling. Only Jeff went. He valued hearing "it was not his fault," that "he wasn't responsible," and that "it wouldn't have to happen to him." He came to believe alcohol had caused his dad's and grandparents' problems and vowed to never drink. He wished Scott had also had therapy. When Scott dropped out of high school, Ray predicted that Jeff would do the same. Unfortunately, Ray died of end-stage cirrhosis the summer Jeff graduated from high school and never knew that his son had matriculated in college. When Ray died of alcoholism, his son Jeff was the same age as Ray had been at Laurence's death.

"I thought you didn't drink," I ventured.

"I didn't. I hated it. But I got stressed and tried a beer, and it relaxed me. I thought I could be like mom and drink to 'take the edge off,' but Dad was right, I was like him—useless."

"How many drinks do you have on an average day?" I asked.

"Sometimes none, sometimes six, sometimes more."

"When did you start drinking more?"

"Last month," he paused. "When Scott was admitted to rehab." Jeff took a breath and continued.

I saw it coming. Scott spun off the road, wound up in the emergency room, and was transferred to the same rehab center Dad had been in.

When I saw Scott, I thought I was looking at Dad. Scott kept yelling, "You'll be like me soon too. It is just a matter of time." That night I drank eight beers to "take the edge off." And now I can't stop. I'm an alcoholic, like Scott and my dad and his dad before him; the whole lot of us are useless. I can't focus at school, and I'm afraid to call Mom; I am all she has left, and I'm a failure.

## The Impact of Alcohol on Health

Different doses of alcohol have different effects on the body. Light to moderate consumption has positive health benefits. Those who drink one to two drinks per day have a lower risk of heart disease, diabetes, stroke, and early mortality overall. This benefit is associated with increases in HDL, decreases in platelet aggregation, and lower plasma fibrinogen concentrations. But more than two drinks per day increases overall mortality rates.[199] Excessive alcohol consumption is the third leading cause of preventable death in the United States, following only smoking and obesity. In males aged fifteen to fifty-nine, alcohol abuse is the single strongest risk factor for premature death. Excessive use of alcohol includes heavy drinking, binge drinking, and drinking while pregnant or underage. Heavy drinking is defined as more than one drink per day on average for women and more than two drinks per day on average for men. Binge drinking is defined as consuming four or more drinks during a single occasion for women and five or more for men. A standard drink, regardless of the variety, contains fourteen grams of ethanol (0.6 fluid ounces of pure alcohol): this includes twelve ounces of beer, five ounces of wine, or one and a half ounces of hard liquor (5 percent, 12 percent, and 40 percent alcohol, respectively).[200]

According to the National Institute on Alcohol Abuse and Alcoholism, genes are responsible for about half of the risk for alcohol-use disorders.[201] Environmental factors determine the additional risk. Roughly 9 percent of American men, 5 percent of women, and 50 percent of college students engage in high-risk drinking. Most people who drink excessively are not alcoholics. But sixteen million Americans meet the diagnostic criteria for alcohol-use disorder, and fewer than 25 percent of those seek and receive formal treatment.[202]

The consequences of excessive drinking are not limited to the alcoholic; families are also severely affected. In general, risks increase with increasing amounts of alcohol. Excessive alcohol use over time increases the risk of consequences of physical, mental, and social health. The following are all associated with excessive or long-term consumption:

- Neurological problems, including dementia, stroke, and neuropathy
- Cardiovascular problems, including myocardial infarction, cardiomyopathy, atrial fibrillation, diabetes, and hypertension
- Psychiatric problems, including depression, anxiety, and suicide
- Social problems, including unemployment, lost productivity, and family problems
- Cancer, including tumors of the mouth, throat, esophagus, liver, colon, and breast
- Liver diseases, including alcoholic hepatitis and cirrhosis
- Other gastrointestinal problems, including pancreatitis, gastritis, and ulcers

The U.S. Preventive Services Task Force recommends screening all adults and providing brief behavioral interventions for those at high risk.[203] The Single Question Screening is a valid instrument for identifying alcohol misuse: "How many times in the past year have you had five (for men) or four (for woman and all adults > 65) or more drinks per day?"[202] An answer of one or more is considered a positive screen and warrants further evaluation. To this one screening question, Jeff answered, "Many." He had not yet experienced tolerance or withdrawal symptoms, but he fitted the criteria for alcohol-use disorder and was at high risk, given his genetics and his environment.

## The Construct of Thoughts from Experiences

Supporters of the nurture-versus-nature model believe we are born with a blank slate or, as John Locke described it, a tabula rasa, with no preconceived ideas, knowledge, or reactions.[204] We have no prejudice, no racism, and no understanding of love or hate until we have experiences and form reactions. We are born with open minds, ready to be molded. In this nurture model, children are receptive to learning, and during the most formative years of life all they know is what they are taught. Once experiences occur, lessons are learned and personal perspectives are formed; we establish a lens through which we view the world. We view life through this subjective window; our lens frames our daily thoughts, feelings, actions, and interactions. All that we do or don't do is based on our reactions to experiences beginning at birth.

## Negativity Bias

"Negativity bias" is consistent with the nurture model and a natural part of evolution that protects us from danger. Stress responses, thoughts, and memories are felt much more strongly in relation to negative experiences than to positive ones.[205] Jonathon Haidt, author of *The Happiness Hypothesis*, explains that we are programmed to respond more strongly to negative than to positive stimuli, as a means of emphasizing details of crucible events to avoid them in the future.[63]

The ability to overcome negative experiences varies by individual and circumstance. When faced with adverse situations, some demonstrate great resilience and bounce back easily; some become permanently limited by irrational and negative thoughts, fears, and behaviors; still others overcome negative thoughts only after a sufficient ratio of positive experiences. John Gottman, a psychologist who researched marital relationships, concluded that "it wasn't only how couples fought that mattered, but how they made up." He described that even in stable marriages, "it takes at least 5 positive actions to overcome one negative action."[206]

Negativity begets negativity and can become irrational, persistent, and destructive. Aaron T. Beck first proposed the theory behind "cognitive distortions" in the 1960s, and David Burns popularized it with common names and examples.[207,208] In 2009 John M. Grohol, PsyD, published "15 Common Cognitive Distortions," a list (reproduced in brief here) of the most common thoughts individuals repeat to themselves that seem rational but are inaccurate distortions of reality and serve only to reinforce negativity.[209]

### 15 COMMON COGNITIVE DISTORTIONS

1. Filtering: an exclusive focus on a single negative aspect of a situation
2. Polarized thinking: a belief that something is all good or all bad, black or white

3. Overgeneralization: a broad conclusion based on a single unpleasant event
4. Jumping to conclusions: a hasty conclusion about how or why someone is behaving as she is
5. Catastrophizing: an expectation that disaster has struck, also referred to as "magnifying"
6. Personalization: a belief that one is alone or at fault for bad outcomes
7. Control fallacies: a sense that one is externally or internally controlled and helpless to influence one's fate
8. Fallacy of fairness: resentment at being treated unfairly
9. Blaming: holding other people responsible for one's outcomes
10. Shoulds: a list of strict rules about how one should behave
11. Emotional reasoning: a conviction that what one feels must automatically be true
12. Fallacy of change: an expectation that other people must change to meet one's personal needs
13. Global labeling: attachment of generalized or unhealthy labels
14. Always being right: an inability to see oneself as being wrong, despite proof or damage to others
15. Heaven's reward fallacy: a belief that self-sacrifice and self-denial pay off

Ray's childhood experience generated several cognitive distortions for him and for his sons. Jeff successfully neutralized many of these by working with therapists. He learned that naming his thoughts promoted understanding and provided the skills to correct his misconceptions. This reframing is consistent with Dr. Grohol's message that "by learning to correctly identify this kind of distorted 'stinkin' thinkin'" a person can then answer the negative thinking back, and refute it. By refuting the negative thinking over and over again, it will slowly diminish over time and be automatically replaced by more rational, balanced thinking."[209]

Jeff's successful coping strategies were lost when he experienced his brother's failings, and they were replaced with negative, irrational self-talk. Jeff was overcome by black-and-white thinking, saying to himself, "I am a failure and always will be." He reverted to viewing life in absolutes—by failing at one thing, he must fail at all. He jumped to conclusions and overgeneralized drinking to his whole identity, claiming, "I can't do anything right," "I'm worthless," and "I'll never amount to anything."

As we accumulate experiences, our core beliefs become solidified, making it challenging to remain open-minded. By the time we are adults, we have collected millions of memories, making it nearly impossible *not* to have thoughts about people, places, and things we encounter. Our personal perspective becomes wired to judge a thing as good or bad, and we develop likes and dislikes, things we approve of and things we don't. Our thoughts have less plasticity, and fixed beliefs form the roots of bias, prejudice, and judgment of others and of ourselves. When this happens, we are paralyzed by our past and must change our story in order not to carry the past into the present and the future.

A full 80 percent of reactions to current situations come not from the situation at hand but from reactions derived from previous experiences. We lay down memories of our learnings and later draw from those to interpret similar or associated experiences. Learnings are collectively harnessed and form the basis for automatic responses to future exposures. Jeff's intense reaction to his brother's drinking was a cumulative response carried over from his experiences with his father.

## The Impact of Experiences, Thoughts, Emotions, and Actions on Outcomes

Experiences, thoughts, emotions, and actions are interrelated in affecting outcomes. Experiences effect our thinking. Thoughts shape how we feel about ourselves, feelings drive our actions, actions influence our interactions with others, and together they determine the outcomes of our performance and our effectiveness in the world. Negative experiences affect pessimistic thinking, drive negative emotions, shape negative actions, and influence negative outcomes. A parallel result holds true for positive thoughts. The process, while appearing linear, is actually continuous, as the outcomes (good or bad) become our next experience.

The Thomas Theorem posits: "That which we believe becomes our real-

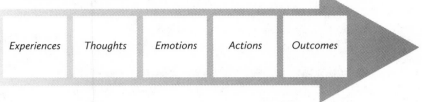

| Experiences | Thoughts | Emotions | Actions | Outcomes |

ity."[210] This theorem is highlighted in a story in which the public believed there to be a shortage of toilet paper, which prompted general fear. The fright drove individuals to purchase excess toilet tissue products, which inevitably created a shortage. This type of self-fulfilling prophecy occurs as thoughts drive bad feelings that we act on in ways that make our thoughts come true. For example, when Jeff believes he is going to fail an exam, he feels hopeless and disillusioned and disengages from studying. He breaks away from academic resources, reverts to isolation and drinking, and thus fails. Unhealthy thought cycles imprison us and limit our ability to change and grow. When we say to ourselves "I can't . . . ," we limit our scope of actions and give away our potential. The Thomas Theorem speaks to the potency of beliefs in shaping reality. It suggests that thoughts drive behaviors in ways consistent with our beliefs, and then our actions enable the narratives we tell ourselves to become reality.

Adverse experiences negatively affect health. The Adverse Childhood Experiences Study demonstrated a direct correlation between negative childhood experiences, high-risk behaviors, and poor health outcomes, including chronic disease and increased overall mortality. Children with the greatest number of adverse experiences demonstrated the highest-risk behaviors and had the worst outcomes. There were exceptions, but the majority of children in alcoholic or abusive homes had unhealthy behaviors and corresponding poor health.[20]

Jeff had insight into the impact of his father's experiences on his father's life, but he didn't see that he also had experienced a destructive environment firsthand. Jeff grew up robbed of a childhood that fostered self-worth. His belief that he was useless caused him to feel defeated, and as a result he drank. Self-destructive behaviors were interwoven with his self-destructive thoughts and feelings. Jeff became unable to reframe his thoughts. He blamed his brother and his father, his anger and fear impelled him to drink, and without support he spiraled downward quickly.

## Reframing Thoughts

We all face challenges every day. Our ability to overcome them depends on how we view them. We can't change past experiences, but we do have the power to change how we interpret them. Changing our interpretation does not mean that we convince ourselves that a bad experience was good; it means that we practice realistic optimism and consider how the situation might look from another's perspective or from a different angle.

At times our thinking is subconscious, and we have automatic negative patterns of thinking that fester. Individuals who call on cognitive flexibility, also sometimes called cognitive reappraisal or cognitive reframing, can change the way they view themselves and the world around them and thus create a new context from which healthy thoughts, feelings, actions, and outcomes can arise. Flexibility in thinking is as important to our health as flexibility in our bodies. Reframing thoughts gives us the power to reverse a cycle away from negative outcomes and toward positive outcomes and a healthier future. Cognitive flexibility is the ability to change maladaptive ruminations. The concept that our thoughts dictate our lives has been in existence for centuries. The Upanishads in the Hindu scriptures states, "What a man thinks upon, he becomes."[211]

Cognitive behavioral therapy (CBT) grew out of the work of Albert Ellis in the 1950s and Aaron T. Beck in the 1960s to prioritize shifting thoughts, as opposed to previous therapy that focused purely on changing maladaptive behaviors.[212,207,213] CBT is a technique that redirects self-destructive thoughts to realign maladaptive behaviors and negative emotions. One of many treatment options used by therapists and providers, CBT can be applied broadly to a range of mental-health conditions, including anxiety, depression, and eating disorders, and can help with sleep difficulties and pain management, as well as addiction treatment.[214] This evidence-based technique is self-directed by patients, in partnership with trained counselors, to tackle deeply ingrained self-defeating, distorted thinking and move toward healthy behavioral patterns. The Beck Institute provides extensive training, and the Academy of Cognitive Therapy (ACT), established in 1998, provides formal certification.[215] CBT is problem-focused, action-oriented, and often short-term, lasting between thirty and ninety days. The CBT model recognizes that past experiences influence thoughts, but, unlike some forms of psychotherapy, it does not dwell on the past, focusing instead on the future. The benefits of CBT include redirecting negative thoughts, regulating unhealthy emotions, correcting maladaptive behaviors, increasing overall resilience to negative experiences, and improving effectiveness in the future.[214] CBT is represented in a triangle, emphasizing the linkage between thoughts, emotions, and behaviors. When any of the three are unhealthy, CBT can be employed to improve health and life.

Core to this approach is a willingness to let go of a strongly held perspective and see a situation from a different angle. CBT framing techniques are used in business and health-care leadership training to transform challenges into opportunities and deliver meaningful personal and professional outcomes.[216,217] Appreciative inquiry, discussed in lesson 2, is a complementary strategy used to focus on positive affirmations and shift away from negative responses. CBT promotes failings as learning opportunities and redirects individuals to seek alternate positive and productive perspectives.

The process of reframing requires identifying thoughts that need changing. Disruptive thoughts might not be obvious until they cause negative consequences. Thus, the reframing process is often initiated after a poor outcome. Individuals work backward from a challenge, to identify associated behaviors, emotions, and thoughts. Specific steps encompass (1) analyzing negative outcomes—specifically, looking at personal thoughts, feelings, and actions that shaped the outcome; (2) recognizing and labeling distorted thoughts; (3) seeking an alternate lens and a positive perspective to achieve healthier thoughts; and (4) affirming these thoughts until previous thoughts are refuted and feelings, behaviors, and outcomes change. The process demands a commitment to honesty about what is not working, and to patience, for practice and transformation take time. The power of negative thoughts to control an individual's actions, and ultimately health, exists in all aspects of an individual's life. Limited thinking shows up in many phrases, including, "I can't," "I have to," "I should," "He can't," and "She should."

Over the next few months I worked with Jeff to deconstruct his negative experiences and consider a new lens, to avoid repeating his father's and brother's patterns. He was fortunate to have had experience in CBT previously, and studied the situation that caused old habits to resurface. Jeff's fears of becoming an alcoholic motivated him to analyze unhealthy behaviors and their origins in his self-defeating thoughts and feelings. In hope of changing his future, he was open to exploring past experiences and how they shaped his thinking, feelings, and actions.

Jeff spoke to his mother, his girlfriend, and his past counselor to negate his misperceptions and to counter messages he received numerous times from his father, such as that he was "useless" and a "loser." Jeff considered different views and gave himself a clean slate. Over several months he journaled and captured the following written affirmations to change his story:

- My dad was an alcoholic, and I took care of him at my own expense.
- My dad's behavior was not excusable but also not incomprehensible, given his own childhood with two alcoholic parents.
- Alcoholism is a disease, and Dad and Scott refused treatment.
- I am not my dad or my brother.
- I finished high school, successfully began college, and want to become a veterinarian.
- I have a track record for drinking moderately.
- My mother is balanced and drinks responsibly, and half my genes come from her.
- My mother loves me, and she will not abandon me.
- I have support from my mother, my girlfriend, and professionals.
- Stress is normal, everyone has it, and it won't kill me.
- I have other ways of coping with stress and "taking the edge off" besides drinking.
- I can take care of myself and not repeat the patterns that I now understand.
- I can take care of myself, as I have done in the past.

Jeff used these affirmations to challenge his thinking and would need to do so continually to direct his life course. He successfully countered nearly all distorted thoughts, but he knew that his default ways of coping could return. Over time he traded his "I can't" self-talk for "I think I can," and later "I can" and "I will." His belief in himself evoked pride and drove success. Success bred confidence, and this positive cycle continued to produce more success. He remained fixed in his all-or-nothing belief about drinking. He wisely chose to not drink. He even attended Alcoholics Anonymous, as his father had refused to do. His mother and girlfriend also abstained from drinking, to show support, and they partnered with him to find alternate strategies to relax. Their support further validated Jeff's decision, his self-worth, and the power of a supportive network.

Our core beliefs in life begin to form as soon as we start to interpret our experiences. Past experiences influence our beliefs, continually feed our thoughts and emotions, and direct our actions. When experiences are interpreted positively, we are effective, balanced, and healthy. But when ingrained patterns are distorted or negative, they limit our abilities. Challenges are universal—everyone experiences them—and when we experience bumps in life, we react. No two people react to an experience identically, but our ability to thrive depends on how we see others, the world, and ourselves. If we view a bump as a mountain, we risk being held hostage to irrational, limiting thoughts. If we consider that same bump to be a part of our journey, we open ourselves up to new ventures and possibilities.

My grandmother was born in 1918 and trained, without college, to be a secretary. When I was accepted to medical school in 1985, the year before she died, she told me that I would make a fabulous doctor. Medicine, she said, was the only profession that would not require writing and would tolerate poor penmanship. I interpreted her simple words as "I am not a writer." I maintained my journal but referred to my notes as just "choppy snippets" of stories. They would "never" become a book, for I believed I was "not a writer." But after sharing my stories, I received different perspectives and positive feedback and came to view my writing as meaningful and beneficial to others. So if you are reading this, you know that I have reframed my thoughts. I now believe that writing has made me a more effective doctor and a healthier person. I am privileged to share what I have learned from and with patients, and I am honored to "be a writer." My grandmother would be surprised and proud.

• ✶ • • • • • • • • ✶ •

HEALTH CHALLENGE #11    Seek an Alternate Lens

The journey of discovering lies not in finding new landscapes,
but in having new eyes.
MARCEL PROUST

This exercise can assist you in looking at an aspect of your life that is not working well and seeking an alternate lens to reframe your story. You have the opportunity to consider the effects of your thoughts on your feelings, actions, and outcomes. Start at the end of the process by identifying a specific outcome in your life that is less than optimal. Work through the following five items to recognize your actions, feelings, and limiting thoughts or cognitive distortions. Last, reframe your thoughts. Review the examples in the table, then rewrite your own story.

1.  Outcomes: Analyze a current challenge or negative outcome. Examine an area of your life—your self-care, relationships, or work or school experience—where you are dissatisfied or less effective than you would like to be. You may review your journal, consider your story from lesson 4, or analyze your time log from lesson 7 or your SMART goal from lesson 9 to find that aspect of your life where you are underperforming or wish to perform better.
2.  Actions: Observe your behaviors. How did your actions shape the outcomes? What feelings triggered your actions?
3.  Feelings: Identify associated feelings. How did your emotions influence your actions? What thoughts triggered your feelings?
4.  Thoughts: Recognize and label any distorted thoughts. What beliefs of yours influenced the situation? Review common distortions and the limiting phrases. Recognize any unhealthy or negative thoughts. Consider the origin of the thoughts. What past experiences contributed to this pattern?

# REFRAMING THOUGHTS TO CHANGE OUTCOMES

| 4. THOUGHTS | 3. FEELINGS | 2. ACTIONS | 1. OUTCOMES | 5. REFRAMED THOUGHTS AND AFFIRMATIONS |
|---|---|---|---|---|
| "I can't . . . relax, communicate, make friends, exercise, lose weight, show my feelings, do anything right, go on like this."<br><br>"I'm not a . . . math person, athlete, writer, speaker, scholar, leader, good traveler, test taker, social person." | Inadequacy<br>Fear<br>Hopelessness<br>Defeat<br>Stupidity<br>Unhealthiness<br>Disempowerment<br>Disappointment<br>Anxiety | Stops trying<br>Stops caring<br>Doesn't apply self<br>Gives up<br>Eats anything<br>Doesn't socialize<br>Remains sedentary<br>Never travels<br>Doesn't vote | Excess drinking<br>Disengagement<br>Weight gain<br>Obesity<br>Heart disease<br>Limited learning<br>Limited potential<br>Limited growth<br>Isolation<br>Loss of purpose | I have an important and unique contribution that can help others.<br><br>I can change.<br><br>I can do anything, when I commit.<br><br>I can improve. |
| I . . . | | | | |
| "I have to, I should . . . do more, be a role model, get a 4.0, like and please everyone, know everything, be less stressed, have the perfect family, take on more, have a better job, be happier."<br><br>I'm too busy and have no time for . . . me, the gym, family, relaxing, reading, friends." | Stress<br>Guilt<br>Inadequacy<br>Exhaustion<br>Frustration<br>Agitation<br>Overwhelm | Never rests<br>Avoids situations<br>Procrastinates | Poor self-image<br>Avoidance<br>Isolation<br>Burnout<br>Self-medication<br>Self-neglect<br>Self-abuse<br>Substance abuse<br>Depression | I'm okay the way I am.<br>I'm not perfect.<br>I am more effective when I do less.<br>I can do what matters to me.<br>I will value the little things I do.<br>I can view time as a gift I give others and myself.<br>I can improve. |
| HE/SHE . . . | | | | |
| "She can't do anything right."<br>"He is a jerk."<br>"She is a racist."<br>"He never listens."<br>"He is annoying." | Blame<br>Anger<br>Distrust | Disrespects self and others<br>Communicates poorly | Isolation<br>Conflict<br>Divided Community<br>Racism<br>Poor team function | I can bring people together by seeing others' strengths.<br>I can find an area we can all agree on.<br>I can respect everyone.<br>I can recognize that everyone struggles. |
| THEY . . . | | | | |
| "They should know better."<br>"They are doing nothing and going nowhere."<br>"Everyone is out for number one."<br>"No one cares about me." | Resentment<br>Anger<br>Distrust<br>Self-righteousness | Doesn't participate if others are not perfect | Disconnection<br>Poor relationships<br>Divisions<br>Prevention of the performance of others | I can listen.<br>I can learn from everyone.<br>I can find value in others' perspectives.<br>I can view everyone as family. |

5. Reframing of thoughts and creation of affirmations: Seek an alternate lens and positive perspectives to challenge the negative thoughts and affirm healthy thoughts. Whom do you trust? Who knows your situation and can offer a different lens or viewpoint? If you are thinking of the worst-case scenario, consider what other possible options exist. Develop a positive and healthy affirmation that you can claim on a daily basis until your habitual thoughts are refuted and feelings, behaviors, and outcomes change. Test your new beliefs on real situations.

• • • • • • • • • • •

# CELEBRATE
# THE JOURNEY

The journey is the reward.

CHINESE PROVERB

I met Sam the week before Mary's first visit. Sam was a colleague who had recently finished her medical training, and she introduced herself as Mary's partner when she came by to drop off their adoption forms. Sam explained how hard the past few years had been and painted a dismal picture of Mary's infertility experience. Sam was thirty-nine but appeared much older. She was businesslike, a bit rushed, but direct; her shirt was pressed, her hair was trimmed meticulously, and she spoke deliberately. She described herself as negative by nature. She was older than most residents and felt the pressure of aging.

Sam described Mary as the person who had changed her life. She considered Mary to be most positive person she knew. Friends since childhood, they shared similar backgrounds and experiences. In the next month she and Mary hoped to travel to Guatemala and return home with a baby. They were in the second round of the adoption process. They had tried unsuccessfully to adopt in Korea.

On Mary's first visit, as with most visits, Sam told their story, but Mary was the one I learned from. Calm and peaceful, Mary was also thirty-nine, yet she appeared to be in her twenties. She flowed as she entered the office, her long curls bouncing and skirt swirling. Mary had married Sam ten years before and had wanted a child ever since. Unsuccessful for over five years at getting pregnant, she was now fully committed to the adoption process.

Mary sat calmly as Sam described their infertility journey. Mary spoke only to convey her excitement at establishing her care with me and one day being a new mother.

For the previous five years their desire for a child had dominated both their lives. Mary had focused primarily on staying healthy and concentrating on her goal. Sam, on the other hand, had been overwhelmed and unable to enjoy the process, her work, or her life. They had been collecting baby clothes, and both desperately wanted to hear a heartbeat on ultrasound. But so far, Sam noted, the only things that grew were the bills and the stress, not a baby.

Sam described how both she and Mary had previously been diagnosed with pelvic inflammatory disease (PID). Both had been treated and retested to confirm that they were cured. Sam recalled how surprisingly pleased Mary had been to have discovered the infection before having children, as she knew the serious complication of chlamydia for newborns. Sam also revealed that Mary had left home at nineteen after being sexually molested by a family member. Mary remarkably saw that experience as a blessing, as it had allowed her to move in with Sam's family. Mary commented on her trauma only to say, "I'm glad it was me and not my sisters, who were so young." Mary was empowered by protecting her siblings. She recognized that the situation was not her fault but that the abuser chose her because she was a "pleaser." She acknowledged that being liked is a good trait, not one that causes rape.

Sam had had a similar experience with sexual assault, by her own stepfather, but she in contrast felt primarily guilt, shame, and disconnection. As a result, she believed that bad things would always happen to her. It wasn't until she learned of Mary's story that she realized that her struggle didn't have to define her. Sam protected Mary, and Mary gave Sam a window into appreciation of herself and others.

## Sexually Transmitted Infections and the Infertility Journey

Sexually transmitted infections (STIs) are public health epidemics that are difficult to identify and track. They also carry great stigma. Over twenty-five diseases are spread primarily through sexual activity. In the United States more than one hundred million individuals are currently living with an STI, and nearly twenty million new cases occur each year, at a health-care cost of over $16 billion annually.[218,219] When I began teaching on this topic in 1999, the prevalence was only sixty-five million and the incidence was twelve million. Rates vary by region and population. The southeastern part of the United States has the highest rates per population. Females are affected more often than males; non-Hispanic blacks represent the highest-risk ethnic group; and 50 percent of new STIs occur in those aged fifteen to twenty-four, although this age represents only 30 percent of the sexually active population.

Chlamydia is particularly widespread among the young, sexually active female population, with 40 percent of cases reported in fifteen- to nineteen-year-olds. Up to 40 percent of women with untreated chlamydia will develop PID, and one in five women with PID will become infertile. Moreover, women infected with PID have a sevenfold increase of ectopic pregnancy and an 18 percent likelihood of having chronic pelvic pain. Women with chlamydia are also three to five times more likely to become infected with HIV, if exposed. In addition, chlamydia causes prematurity, eye disease, and pneumonia in infants. The U.S. Preventive Services Task Force and CDC recommend screening all sexually active women under age twenty-five for chlamydia but have found insufficient evidence to warrant screening males. Diagnosis can be made with new DNA methods, which offer high sensitivity and a specificity not achieved with older tests. The CDC's 2015 treatment guidelines recommended single-dose treatment, which can also be used during pregnancy, to increase compliance, but it is insufficient if PID develops.[218,220,221]

Infertility is a complex issue. It can have numerous causes, stemming from a female or male partner. Artificial insemination began in the 1970s and has been a valuable procedure for those, including couples who are infertile, wishing to rely on a sperm donor; single women; and same-sex couples. Artificial insemination is an advanced fertilization procedure in which sperm is artificially placed, through introduction of a thin, flexible tube, in a woman's cervix (intracervical insemination) or uterus (intrauterine insemination). The procedure is considered safe and painless, but the rate of becoming pregnant varies by the female's age, the reason for procedure, and the potential causes of infertility. Rates range from 5 percent to 25 percent with each menstrual cycle and increase when fertility drugs are taken in conjunction with the procedure.

In vitro fertilization (IVF), first carried out in England in 1978, became available in the United States in 1981. Nearly two hundred thousand babies have been born in the United States thanks to IVF. Babies resulting from this procedure were initially labeled test-tube babies, since the embryo forms in a laboratory, outside the human body. The procedure is more complex and costly than artificial insemination. It takes place in cycles, with detailed attention paid to accommodating the timing of the female ovulatory cycle and hormonal levels. With ultrasound guidance, a mature egg is removed with a fine needle from a follicle in the ovary, while the patient is on pain medication or under sedation. Eggs are fertilized by a sperm in vitro and placed back in the uterus a few days later for the nine-month gestation period. The National Infertility Association reports that pregnancy occurs nearly 30 percent of the time; a live birth results in approximately 20 percent of all cases. Age is a major factor in the outcome of the procedure. Patients older than forty have rates as low as 10 percent by comparison with those under thirty-five, whose rates can be as high as 40 percent. A single cycle can cost upward of $12,000. The National Infertility Association publishes a booklet called the *Infertility Insurance Advisor*, which provides tips on insurance benefits.[222]

Mary and Sam had both grown up in Vermont, and Mary expressed how grateful she had been when they were able to get a civil union in 2000. When they moved to Massachusetts in 2003 to marry, Mary had already identified a sperm donor, and they had agreed to begin the process of artificial insemination. When Vermont passed legislation permitting them to marry legally, they moved back home in 2009. Mary also expressed how grateful she was that the United States, unlike some other countries (such as Switzerland, Germany, or Hong Kong), did not restrict artificial insemination to heterosexual couples. She had known how much money the process could cost and had been thankful for every penny they earned and saved to support a child. Sam, on the other hand, had worried they would have no money left to raise the child or, worse yet, have nothing to show for what they spent.

When Mary had begun the intrauterine insemination process, she was thirty-four and was given an estimated 5 percent to 25 percent likelihood of pregnancy. She watched her temperature like a hawk, documented her cycles, had regular ultrasounds, and had blood drawn to predict the exact day, if not moment, she would ovulate. They drew so much blood that Sam had feared that Mary would become anemic, but Mary viewed the process as simple and was happy to monitor her cycles. She had enjoyed plotting out the dates and guessing the baby's birthday with each attempt. Mary kept a running list of potential birthdays for potential children and continued to knit a baby blanket and anticipate celebrating that special day.

Sam explained that after artificial insemination was unsuccessful, an exhaustive workup revealed extensive scarring on Mary's fallopian tubes. Surgery and an additional attempt at artificial insemination did not result in a child. Sam was prepared to accept the fact that a child was not in their future. She herself did not wish to become pregnant, but Mary wished to move forward with IVF. She knew that IVF was more time-consuming, complex, and expensive, but she wanted to try it. Mary viewed the IVF time commitment as an extended opportunity to honor and care for herself: no drinking, medication, or smoking, and continual healthy eating, exercise, and sleep. As she underwent more testing, blood work, hormone injections, ultrasounds, and appointments, she tracked all of these in her baby book, like milestones in a child's development. She continued to calculate the "estimated date of confinement," based on her last menstrual period, as a potential birthday for a future child.

Sam told us how Mary's first IVF cycle failed, as did her second and her third. As Mary aged, she knew, her likelihood of success diminished. Sam was ready to throw in the towel many times over, but Mary was thankful for the extra time. She believed that when she finally became a mother and her child arrived, they would all be ready. I completed Mary's physical exam and their application forms. Mary thanked me for participating in this special time in her life and asked if I would be the baby's doctor as well. If all went well, they would be back from Guatemala and scheduling a newborn well-child visit soon.

## The Benefits of Gratitude

Gratitude, the focus of much research, increases health and happiness. The act of celebrating is an active expression of appreciation. Deborah Norville, author of *Thank You Power: Making the Science of Gratitude Work for You*, summarized studies showing that those who practiced gratitude exercised more, had fewer illnesses, got more sleep, and experienced decreased anxiety and depression.[223] Benefits occurred independent of economic status, race, gender, or religion. Appreciation is an expression of optimism and fosters positive emotions. Dr. Barbara Fredrickson, a psychologist at the University of North Carolina, researched positive emotions and their relation to "biological markers of health" and concluded that their effect was to "lower levels of stress-related hormones" and increase "dopamine and opioids [which enhance] immune system functioning and [diminish] inflammatory responses to stress."[224] Being appreciative also makes people less envious and more secure, determined, optimistic, energetic, and enthusiastic. Grateful individuals are better able to handle challenges and are more satisfied with life.

Appreciation, like many strategies discussed in this book, is a simple concept but is not always easily achieved. Life's journey guarantees stresses. Some of them, such as a viral illness, are short-lived, but some stresses stay with us for life, such as the loss of a child or a disability due to depression. A full 90 percent of individuals will experience at least one major traumatic event in their lifetime.[7,225] Reflecting on Mary and other patients, I am reminded that everyone I meet is struggling with something in his or her life. Gratitude is a strategy for adapting to those challenges, one based on the concept that no matter how difficult life is at any point, there is always something for which to be grateful. Mary's appreciative outlook on life benefited her and Sam. As Oprah claimed in her recent book, *What I Know for Sure*, "The more grateful you become, the more you have to be grateful for."[226]

Life is often a circuitous path, with twists and turns that can affect health. Reframing obstacles as learning opportunities, valuing individual steps toward a goal, and acknowledging the joy of ordinary things are the basis for appreciation and celebration. Life is richest and health is optimal when we face challenges, move progressively forward, and value the treasures we possess every day.

## Celebrate Challenges

Celebrating challenges is not about idealizing a problem but about seeing value in overcoming problems. Failings are potent prompts for both reflecting on what is not currently working and for reviewing what has worked in the past. Adverse events, if we can appreciate them, are points of maximum learning, and by rejoicing in our capacity to learn, no matter how uncomfortable we get, we have plenty to celebrate.

There is more to success than external achievement. The greatest potential for internal growth exists in overcoming personal challenges. Each test in life has the potential to build internal character. We are given one chance at life, and the ability to become unstuck when something goes awry is a skill worthy of revelry. When your flight is canceled, how do you respond to being stuck in the Philadelphia airport? Does your reaction escalate stress and set a harsh tone for the trip, or can you adjust and say, "That's okay. I get more time now with my family to have a nice dinner." I couldn't help but appreciate and celebrate my daughter's wisdom when during a recent layover she used those exact words.

Mary excelled at celebrating challenges; she allowed each bump to make her a better person and future parent. She worshipped time spent reflecting and celebrated the knowledge she gained from her journey. She appreciated that her career as a writer was flexible, and she saw Sam's overwhelming job as a means of easing their access to health resources. She was thankful that past infections had affected only her body and not her mind or spirit. Mary was proud of what she could do and learned from what she couldn't do.

## Celebrate Progress

In addition to celebrating challenges, we can view each and every step toward large achievements as a minisuccess. Life is a long-term investment, and if we embrace the glory of our impermanence, we can enjoy the journey. We don't need to wait for the whole; celebrating the sum of the parts can be superior. Jonathan Haidt, in his book *The Happiness Hypothesis*, presented the progress principle by acknowledging that "pleasure comes more from making progress toward goals than from achieving them." He advised readers "to feel the pleasure as you walk, and not wait for the thrill of removing the backpack at the end of a long hike."[63]

Celebrating along a difficult path can be motivating. I may not have completely achieved my project or even a single goal, but taking a difficult step in the right direction is cause to pause and tell myself, "I have more work to do, but I did a great job getting to where I am now." Doing so is rejuvenating, particularly when there is far to go. Patients who recognize their own progress are motivated to move toward goals. Mary excelled at celebrating her progress. She was at peace with the long hauls of IVF and adoption. She viewed herself as the luckiest women alive because her pregnancy experience lasted five-plus years. With each day she felt better prepared to be a parent, knowing that each step taught her something new about life.

## Celebrate the Day-to-Day Things

Great achievements in life should be recognized: births, graduations, weddings, and promotions. But waiting for these big moments doesn't mean neglecting to honor small wins that make up the majority of our moments. Don't wait for your birthday; turn ordinary experiences into life's treasures. Small wins add up! We can count on everyday rituals to bring us joy. Most Americans give thanks on the third Thursday of November—Thanksgiving Day. But many fail to appreciate all that they have day to day. By incorporating appreciation into a daily practice, we are less likely to move too fast, feel dissatisfied, or take for granted the gifts we have been given.

Dr. Fredrickson referred to "micro moments of positivity," which are defined as "repeated brief moments of positive feelings [that] can provide a buffer against stress and depression and foster both physical and mental health."[224] She also highlighted the importance of activating these purposeful positive experiences to counter normal or excessive negative emotions and suggested an ideal ratio of 3:1 positive to negative.[227] So depending on our daily experiences, we may need more or less celebrating.

After meeting Mary and Sam, and reflecting on Mary's appreciative way, I expanded my habit of living in the spirit of gratitude by appreciating and celebrating simple day-to-day things. I began asking patients what they were thankful for and what they celebrated in their lives. Specific names of people—relatives and friends—were the most common answers I heard. It gave me pause to think about the little things in my life, and what I would miss if they went away. The first is my Earl Grey tea, which I enjoy on the porch every morning in the summer and in the kitchen the rest of the year. The second is my journal, and the third is my daily time to reflect and walk my dog.

Working with different socioeconomic groups and diverse cultures across the United States, as well as in Thailand, China, South Africa, Honduras, and Nicaragua, I have noted that, it paradoxically appears easier for those who have less to appreciate more. Appreciation is not linked to quantity. The U.S. culture values stuff: stuff to put in homes and decorate bodies, stuff to add to résumés, hang on walls, and impress others. Sometimes stuff adds work and not joy: another pair of shoes to polish or shirt to press or achievement to distract us from living life the way we deem important. External stuff can prevent us from being internally focused. This doesn't mean that things can't provide joy, but there is a tipping point at which the accumulation of stuff zaps our attention and limits our appreciation. Chaperoning a service trip to Nicaragua, I observed high school students' shock at seeing extreme poverty juxtaposed with enormous joy. For many of these privileged students, it was their first exposure to and appreciation of the concept "less is more."

I also ask patients how they show their appreciation to others and themselves. Just as there is not one way to optimize health, there is no single way to celebrate our lives. The most commonly shared way of showing thanks has been the spoken word. "I tell people every day how much I value and love them." A few still write letters. "I write old fashioned cards when I want to thank someone." Many consider time the greatest gift they give; others give presents or experiences. I often use my journal as a way to thank myself. I reread entries to see where I added value or to congratulate me.

Mary celebrated many day-to-day things; she didn't just wait for birthdays to celebrate. She kept her life simple, allowing herself time to appreciate ordinary happenings: a good night's sleep, the baby blanket she'd knitted, time for writing. Two months later, Mary and Sam returned from Guatemala, with baby Joy. Mary was ecstatic and had named the baby for the belief that everything in her world is connected. Mary was told that the baby's birthday was not clearly documented. That seemed an irony, given how many possible birthdays she had held sacred. Mary knitted the date March 12 on the baby blanket, but she and Sam agreed to celebrate Joy every day.

## Celebrating a Doctor's Dozen

The impact we all have on society depends not just on our ability to contribute to others but on our ability to prioritize self-care, sustain personal well-being, and model wellness. As health professionals, we have long been revered for our dedication to the health of others, but we cannot afford poor health ourselves. We can and must address this individually and systematically. It is within the power of all of us to know ourselves, to care for ourselves, and—when needed—to improve ourselves. By advancing our own health, we better our lives and the lives of others.

The goal is not perfection, but continual personal growth and development. As I reflect on the lessons, strategies, and stories included here, I continue to observe myself and others, ask questions, reflect on my resilience, and journal my story. I am grateful as I strive for balance in eating, sleeping, exercising, and preserving time for others and myself. I am thankful even when struggling, as I am prompted to pursue authentic and healthy choices; change my thoughts, feelings, and actions; and celebrate that which is positive in my health and my life.

• ✦ ● ● ▶ ● ● ● ● ✦ ●

HEALTH CHALLENGE #12    Practice Gratitude

There is just one life for each of us: our own.

EURIPIDES

The final health challenge is to actively celebrate your progress toward personal wellness. Reflect on the first question, while considering struggles and successes you have faced in each of the health challenges, including your personal health–improvement tool (PHIT). For the second question, identify ways to celebrate your health and practice gratitude each day.

1. Reflect on your challenges, progress, and day-to-day treasures, to identify reasons to celebrate.
   a. Challenges: What did you face today that provided you an opportunity to learn? What are you struggling with that can promote your growth?
   b. Progress: What steps toward personal health improvement are you most proud of? What have you done to foster your ability to be mindful? To ask questions? To build resilience? To practice

self-reflection? To fill your own tank? To practice self-care? To strengthen a relationship? To focus your time on your priorities? To be a role model? To change a behavior? To make a healthy choice? To reframe your thinking?

    c. Day-to-Day Treasures:

- From what or whom did you get joy today?
- Whom and what are you most thankful for?
- What do you love about yourself, your family, your work, your home?
- What did you do well today?

2. Do one thing today and every day to celebrate your health and your life.

    a. Add an appreciation entry to your daily journal.

    b. Send a note of gratitude to yourself or someone you value.

    c. Turn to your neighbors and thank them for working so hard.

    d. Have a party to celebrate your strengths.

    e. Create an award to honor your or someone else's skills.

    f. Invite a friend to dinner to recognize your relationship.

    g. Acknowledge someone who has contributed to your life.

# ACKNOWLEDGMENTS

I am most grateful to all my patients, mentors, and mentees for committing to my health, their health, and the health of our community. I wish to celebrate:

My mother, who loves all for their strengths and accepts without judging.

My father, whose strength of mind and body taught me that to struggle was to build character.

My brothers, who have always protected, guided, and inspired me.

My extended family, who have shared their learnings on life's journey.

My husband, who represents the best choice I have made in my life and who, purposefully, chose me.

Stephanie, my insightful eighteen-year-old, who smells all the roses and continually keeps a clean slate.

Victoria, my mature twenty-one-year-old, who loves to learn and keeps her Nikes on, ready to "just do it."

Evelyn Rosario, my childhood friend and mentor, who was born knowing all that I learned in five decades.

Linda Patchet, for reminding me to breathe before, during, and after budget meetings and for introducing me and our team to the "Word of the Year."

Pam Gile, who left me her appreciation for every second, of every moment, of every day.

Members of my "Team," who keep their integrity and their commitments to themselves and one another.

Kathryn Patton, Kristin Knutzen and Jason Beaton, who helped design and disseminate www.myphit.org.

Deborah Heimann, Jenny Blue, and Drs. Stanley Kozakowski, Joseph Scherger, and Robert Santulli, who inspired me by generously reading and providing invaluable feedback on life and every word of this book.

Phyllis Deutsch, Richard Pult, Susan Abel, and Susan Silver, my editors, who believed in my message and compelled me to write succinctly.

The entire UPNE team for your time, expertise, and commitment to authors and readers; your work lives on forever.

You, my reader, for committing to your own health and to the health of others.

# REFERENCES

1. Jaffe HW, Frieden TR. Improving health in the USA: Progress and challenges. *Lancet.* 2014;384(9937):3–5.
2. World life expectency. Centers for Disease Control and Prevention. 2014; www.worldlifeexpectancy.com. Accessed May 29, 2017.
3. Turnock BJ. *Public Health: What It Is and How It Works.* 5th ed. Burlington, MA: Jones and Bartlett Learning; 2012.
4. Constitution of WHO: Principles. World Health Organization. 1946; www.who.int/en/. Accessed May 28, 2017.
5. Naci H, Ioannidis JP. Evaluation of wellness determinants and interventions by citizen scientists. *JAMA.* 2015;314(2):121–122.
6. Moyer VA. Screening and behavioral counseling interventions in primary care to reduce alcohol misuse: U.S. Preventive Services Task Force recommendation statement. *Annals of Internal Medicine.* 2013;159(3):210–218.
7. Southwick SM, Charney DS. *Resilience: The Science of Mastering Life's Greatest Challenges.* New York, NY: Cambridge University Press; 2012.
8. Koenig HG, Pearce MJ, Nelson B, et al. Effects of religious versus standard cognitive-behavioral therapy on optimism in persons with major depression and chronic medical illness *Depression and Anxiety.* 2015;32(11):835–842.
9. Religious Landscape Study. Pew Research Center. 2014; www.pewforum.org. Accessed May 29, 2017.
10. Cacioppo JT, Cacioppo S. Older adults reporting social isolation or loneliness show poorer cognitive function 4 years later. *Evidence-Based Nursing.* 2014;17(2):59–60.
11. Uchino BN, Cacioppo JT, Kiecolt-Glaser JK. The relationship between social support and physiological processes: A review with emphasis on underlying mechanisms and implications for health. *Psychological Bulletin.* 1996;199(3):488–531.
12. Yang YC, Boen C, Gerken K, et al. Social relationships and physiological determinants of longevity across the human life span. *Proceedings of the National Academy of Sciences of the United States of America.* 2016;113(3):578–583.
13. Cole SW, Capitanio JP, Chun K, et al. Myeloid differentiation architecture of leukocyte transcriptome dynamics in perceived social isolation.

Proceedings of the National Academy of Sciences of the United States of America. 2015;112(49):15142–15147.

14. Rosen LD. *iDisorder: Understanding Our Obsession with Technology and Overcoming Its Hold on Us.* New York, NY: St. Martin's Press; 2013.

15. Brody JE. Hooked on our smartphones. *New York Times.* January 9, 2017.

16. Marmot M. *The Status Syndrome: How Social Standing Affects Our Health and Longevity.* New York, NY: Owl Books/Holt; 2005.

17. Shanafelt TD, Hasan O, Dyrbye LN, et al. Changes in burnout and satisfaction with work-life balance in physicians and the general US working population between 2011 and 2014. *Mayo Clinic Proceedings.* 2015;90(12):1600–1613.

18. Leiter MP, Maslach C. Six areas of worklife: A model of the organizational context of burnout. *Journal of Health and Human Services Administration.* 1999;21(4):472–489.

19. Capaldi CA, Passmore H-A, Nisbet EK, et al. Flourishing in nature: A review of the benefits of connecting with nature and its application as a wellbeing intervention. *International Journal of Wellbeing.* 2015;5(4):1–16.

20. Felitti VJ, Anda RF, Nordenberg D, et al. Relationship of childhood abuse and household dysfunction to many of the leading causes of death in adults. Adverse Childhood Experiences (ACE) Study. *American Journal of Preventive Medicine.* 1998;14(4):245–258.

21. Yerkes RM, Dodson JD. The study of human behavior. *Science.* 1914;39(1009):625–633.

22. Maslach C, Schaufeli WB, Leiter MP. Job burnout. *Annual Review of Psychology.* 2001;52:397–422.

23. Kearney MK, Weininger RB, Vachon ML, et al. Self-care of physicians caring for patients at the end of life: "Being connected . . . a key to my survival." *JAMA.* 2009;301(11):1155–1164, e1151.

24. Davis S, Lind BK, Sorensen C. A comparison of burnout among oncology nurses working in adult and pediatric inpatient and outpatient settings. *Oncology Nursing Forum.* 2013;40(4):E303–311.

25. Slavin SJ. Medical student mental health: Culture, environment, and the need for change. *JAMA.* 2016;316(21):2195–2196.

26. Dyrbye LN, West CP, Satele D, et al. Burnout among U.S. medical students, residents, and early career physicians relative to the general U.S. population. *Academic Medicine: Journal of the Association of American Medical Colleges.* 2014;89(3):443–451.

27. Holleman WL, Cofta-Woerpel LM, Gritz ER. Stress and morale of academic biomedical scientists. *Academic medicine: Journal of the Association of American Medical Colleges.* 2015;90(5):562–564.

28. Livingston M, Livingston H. Emotional distress in nurses at work. *British Journal of Medical Psychology.* 1984;57(Pt.3):291–294.

29. Aiken LH, Clarke SP, Sloane DM, et al. Nurses' reports on hospital care in five countries. *Health Affairs (Millwood).* 2001;20(3):43–53.

30. Dyrbye LN, Varkey P, Boone SL, et al. Physician satisfaction and burnout at different career stages. *Mayo Clinic Proceedings.* 2013;88(12):1358–1367.

31. Dyrbye LN, Satele D, Sloan J, et al. Ability of the physician well-being index to identify residents in distress. *Journal of Graduate Medical Education.* 2014;6(1):78–84.

32. Wurm W, Vogel K, Holl A, et al. Depression-burnout overlap in physicians. *PLOS One.* 2016;11(3):e0149913.

33. Van der Heijden F, Dillingh G, Bakker A, et al. Suicidal thoughts among medical residents with burnout. *Archives of Suicide Research.* 2008;12(4): 344–346.

34. Shanafelt TD, Balch CM, Bechamps GJ, et al. Burnout and career satisfaction among American surgeons. *Annals of Surgury.* 2009;250(3):463–471.

35. Rotenstein LS, Ramos MA, Torre M, et al. Prevalence of depression, depressive symptoms, and suicidal ideation among medical students: A systematic review and meta-analysis. *JAMA.* 2016;316(21):2214–2236.

36. Dewa CS, Loong D, Bonato S, et al. How does burnout affect physician productivity? A systematic literature review. *BMC Health Services Research.* 2014;14:325.

37. Dewa CS, Jacobs P, Thanh NX, et al. An estimate of the cost of burnout on early retirement and reduction in clinical hours of practicing physicians in Canada. *BMC Health Services Research.* 2014;14:254.

38. Shanafelt TD, Mungo M, Schmitgen J, et al. Longitudinal study evaluating the association between physician burnout and changes in professional work effort. *Mayo Clinic Proceedings.* 2016;91(4):422–431.

39. Dyrbye LN, Shanafelt TD. Physician burnout: A potential threat to successful health care reform. *JAMA.* 2011;305(19):2009–2010.

40. Panagioti M, Panagopoulou E, Bower P, et al. Controlled interventions to reduce burnout in physicians: A systematic review and meta-analysis. *JAMA Internal Medicine.* 2017;177(2):195–205.

41. Ratanawongsa N, Roter D, Beach MC, et al. Physician burnout and patient-physician communication during primary care encounters. *Journal of General Internal Medicine.* 2008;23(10):1581–1588.

42. West CP, Huschka MM, Novotny PJ, et al. Association of perceived medical errors with resident distress and empathy: A prospective longitudinal study. *JAMA.* 2006;296(9):1071–1078.

43. West CP, Tan AD, Habermann TM, et al. Association of resident fatigue and distress with perceived medical errors. *JAMA*. 2009;302(12):1294–1300.

44. Fahrenkopf AM, Sectish TC, Barger LK, et al. Rates of medication errors among depressed and burnt out residents: prospective cohort study. *British Medical Journal (Clinical Research Edition)*. 2008;336(7642):488–491.

45. Shanafelt TD, Balch CM, Bechamps G, et al. Burnout and medical errors among American surgeons. *Annals of Surgury*. 2010;251(6):995–1000.

46. Sanchez-Reilly S, Morrison LJ, Carey E, et al. Caring for oneself to care for others: Physicians and their self-care. *Journal of Supportive Oncology*. 2013;11(2):75–81.

47. Shanafelt TD, Boone S, Tan L, et al. Burnout and satisfaction with work-life balance among US physicians relative to the general US population. *Archives of Internal Medicine*. 2012;172(18):1377–1385.

48. Shanafelt TD, Sloan JA, Habermann TM. The well-being of physicians. *American Journal of Medicine*. 2003;114(6):513–519.

49. Plato. *Plato in Twelve Volumes*. Cambridge, MA: Harvard University Press; London, UK: Heinemann; 1969.

50. Gino F, Staats B. Why organizations don't learn. *Harvard Business Review*. November 2015.

51. Brazeau CM, Shanafelt T, Durning SJ, et al. Distress among matriculating medical students relative to the general population. *Academic Medicine: Journal of the Association of American Medical Colleges*. 2014;89(11):1520–1525.

52. Bodenheimer T, Sinsky C. From triple to quadruple aim: Care of the patient requires care of the provider. *Annals of Family Medicine*. 2014;12(6):573–576.

53. Wasson LT, Cusmano A, Meli L, et al. Association between learning environment interventions and medical student well-being: A systematic review. *JAMA*. 2016;316(21):2237–2252.

54. Peterson U, Bergstrom G, Samuelsson M, et al. Reflecting peer-support groups in the prevention of stress and burnout: Randomized controlled trial. *Journal of Advanced Nursing*. 2008;63(5):506–516.

55. Shanafelt TD, Noseworthy JH. Executive leadership and physician well-being: Nine organizational strategies to promote engagement and reduce burnout. *Mayo Clinic Proceedings*. 2017;92(1):129–146.

56. West CP, Dyrbye LN, Erwin PJ, et al. Interventions to prevent and reduce physician burnout: A systematic review and meta-analysis. *Lancet*. 2016;388(10057):2272–2281.

57. Luckiest man. National Baseball Hall of Fame. 1939; https://baseballhall.org . Accessed November 28, 2017.

58. Epstein RM. Mindful practice. *JAMA*. 1999;282(9):833–839.

59. Kabat-Zinn J. *Wherever You Go, There You Are: Mindfulness Meditation in Everyday Life.* New York, NY: Hyperion; 1994.

60. Carlson LE, Brown KW. Validation of the Mindful Attention Awareness Scale in a cancer population. *Journal of Psychosomatic Research.* 2005;58(1):29–33.

61. Hurley D. Breathing in vs. spacing out. *New York Times Magazine.* January 14, 2014.

62. Fjorback LO, Arendt M, Ornbol E, et al. Mindfulness-based stress reduction and mindfulness-based cognitive therapy: A systematic review of randomized controlled trials. *Acta Psychiatrica Scandinavica.* 2011;124(2):102–119.

63. Haidt J. *The Happiness Hypothesis: Finding Modern Truth in Ancient Wisdom.* New York, NY: Basic Books; 2006.

64. McEwen BS. Physiology and neurobiology of stress and adaptation: Central role of the brain. *Physiological Reviews.* 2007;87(3):873–904.

65. Ricard M, Lutz A, Davidson RJ. Mind of the meditator. *Scientific American.* 2014;311(5):38–45.

66. Varela FJ, Thompson E, Rosch E. *The Embodied Mind: Cognitive Science and Human Experience.* Cambridge, MA: MIT Press; 1991.

67. Khoury B, Lecomte T, Fortin G, et al. Mindfulness-based therapy: A comprehensive meta-analysis. *Clinical Psychology Review.* 2013;33(6):763–771.

68. Ludwig DS, Kabat-Zinn J. Mindfulness in medicine. *JAMA.* 2008;300(11):1350–1352.

69. Carlson LE, Speca M, Patel KD, et al. Mindfulness-based stress reduction in relation to quality of life, mood, symptoms of stress, and immune parameters in breast and prostate cancer outpatients. *Psychosomatic Medicine.* 2003;65(4):571–581.

70. Carlson LE, Speca M, Patel KD, et al. Mindfulness-based stress reduction in relation to quality of life, mood, symptoms of stress and levels of cortisol, dehydroepiandrosterone sulfate (DHEAS) and melatonin in breast and prostate cancer outpatients. *Psychoneuroendocrinology.* 2004;29(4):448–474.

71. Carlson LE, Ursuliak Z, Goodey E, et al. The effects of a mindfulness meditation-based stress reduction program on mood and symptoms of stress in cancer outpatients: 6-month follow-up. *Supportive Care in Cancer: Official Journal of the Multinational Association of Supportive Care in Cancer.* 2001;9(2):112–123.

72. Grossman P, Niemann L, Schmidt S, et al. Mindfulness-based stress reduction and health benefits. A meta-analysis. *Journal of Psychosomatic Research.* 2004;57(1):35–43.

73. Speca M, Carlson LE, Goodey E, et al. A randomized, wait-list controlled

clinical trial: The effect of a mindfulness meditation-based stress reduction program on mood and symptoms of stress in cancer outpatients. *Psychosomatic Medicine.* 2000;62(5):613–622.

74. Langer EJ. *The Power of Mindful Learning.* Boston, MA: Da Capo; 1997.

75. Bohlmeijer E, Prenger R, Taal E, et al. The effects of mindfulness-based stress reduction therapy on mental health of adults with a chronic medical disease: A meta-analysis. *Journal of Psychosomatic Research.* 2010;68(6):539–544.

76. Lauche R, Cramer H, Dobos G, et al. A systematic review and meta-analysis of mindfulness-based stress reduction for the fibromyalgia syndrome. *Journal of Psychosomatic Research.* 2013;75(6):500–510.

77. Zgierska A, Rabago D, Chawla N, et al. Mindfulness meditation for substance use disorders: A systematic review. *Substance Abuse.* 2009;30(4):266–294.

78. Fortney L, Luchterhand C, Zakletskaia L, et al. Abbreviated mindfulness intervention for job satisfaction, quality of life, and compassion in primary care clinicians: A pilot study. *Annals of Family Medicine.* 2013;11(5):412–420.

79. Krasner MS, Epstein RM, Beckman H, et al. Association of an educational program in mindful communication with burnout, empathy, and attitudes among primary care physicians. *JAMA.* 2009;302(12):1284–1293.

80. Beach MC, Roter D, Korthuis PT, et al. A multicenter study of physician mindfulness and health care quality. *Annals of Family Medicine.* 2013;11(5):421–428.

81. Nhất Hạnh T. *The Pocket Thich Nhất Hạnh.* Compiled and edited by Melvin McLeod. Boston, MA: Shambala 2012.

82. Nhất Hạnh T. *The Miracle of Mindfulness: An Introduction to the Practice of Mindfulness Translated by Mobi Ho.* Boston, MA: Beacon; 1975.

83. Suzuki S. *Zen Mind, Beginner's Mind: Informal Talks on Zen Meditation and Practice.* Boston, MA: Shambhala; 2011.

84. Covey SR. *The 7 Habits of Highly Effective People: Powerful Lessons in Personal Change.* New York, NY: Simon and Schuster; 2004.

85. Reid TR. *Confucius Lives Next Door: What Living in the East Teaches Us about Living in The West.* New York, NY: Random House; 1999.

86. Byock I. *Dying Well: Peace and Possibilities at the End of Life.* New York, NY: Berkley; 1998.

87. Byock I. *The Four Things That Matter Most: A Book about Living.* New York, NY: Atria Books; 2004.

88. Hawthorne N. *The Birth-Mark.* Boston, MA: Pioneer; 1843.

89. De Voltaire FMA. *The Portable Voltaire.* New York, NY: Viking Penquin; 1949.

90. Native American legends: Two wolves. First People: The Legends. www.firstpeople.us. Accessed May 29, 2017.

91. Boylan JF. *She's Not There: A Life in Two Genders.* New York, NY: Broadway Books; 2003.

92. Haas AP, Eliason M, Mays VM, et al. Suicide and suicide risk in lesbian, gay, bisexual, and transgender populations: Review and recommendations. *Journal of Homosexuality.* 2011;58(1):10–51.

93. Hatzenbuehler ML, Bellatorre A, Lee Y, et al. Structural stigma and all-cause mortality in sexual minority populations. *Social Science and Medicine.* 2014;103:33–41.

94. Russell ST, Joyner K. Adolescent sexual orientation and suicide risk: Evidence from a national study. *American Journal of Public Health.* 2001;91(8):1276–1281.

95. Warning signs of suicide. Trevor Project. www.thetrevorproject.org. Accessed December 7, 2017.

96. Baker K, Garcia J. National Action Alliance for Suicide Prevention tackles LGBT suicide. *National Action Alliance for Suicide Prevention.* April 26, 2012.

97. Rich CL, Fowler RC, Young D, et al. San Diego suicide study: Comparison of gay to straight males. *Suicide and Life-Threatening Behavior.* 1986;16(4): 448–457.

98. Bagley C, Tremblay P. Elevated rates of suicidal behavior in gay, lesbian, and bisexual youth. *Crisis.* 2000;21(3):111–117.

99. Johnson RB, Oxendine S, Taub DJ, et al. Suicide prevention for LGBT students. *New Directions for Student Services.* 2013;2013(141):55–69.

100. Simone MJ, Appelbaum JS. Addressing the needs of older lesbian, gay, bisexual, and transgender adults. *Clinical Geriatrics.* 2011;19(2):38–45.

101. Ryan C, Russell ST, Huebner D, et al. Family acceptance in adolescence and the health of LGBT young adults. *Journal of Child and Adolescent Psychiatric Nursing.* 2010;23(4):205–213.

102. Walls NE, Wisneski H, Kane S. School climate, individual support, or both? Gay straight alliances and the mental health of sexual minority youth. *School Social Work Journal.* 2013;37(2):88–111.

103. Baker KE. The future of transgender coverage. *New England Journal of Medicine.* 2017;376(19):1801–1804.

104. Hyderi A, Angel J, Madison M, et al. Transgender patients: Providing sensitive care. *Journal of Family Practice.* 2016;65(7):450–461.

105. Kübler-Ross E, Kessler D. *On Grief and Grieving: Finding the Meaning of Grief through the Five Stages of Loss.* New York, NY: Scribner; 2005.

106. Grant JM, Mottet LA, Tanis J, et al. *National Transgender Discrimination Survey Report on Health and Health Care.* Washington, DC: National Center for Transgender Equality; October 2010.

107. Ellison R. *Invisible Man.* New York, NY: Vintage International; 1995.

108. The road to resilience. American Psychological Association. 2017; www.apa. org. Accessed May 29, 2017.

109. Coutu D. How resilience works. *Harvard Business Review*. May 2002.

110. Garmezy N. Resilience in children's adaptation to negative life events and stressed environments. *Pediatric Annals*. 1991;20(9):459–460, 463–456.

111. Werner EE. What can we learn about resilience from large-scale longitudinal studies? In: Goldstein S, Brooks R, eds. *Handbook of Resilience in Children*. Boston, MA: Springer; 2013.

112. Dugard J. *Freedom: My Book of Firsts*. New York, NY: Simon and Schuster; 2016.

113. Nielson S. How to survive solitary confinement. *Psychology*. January 28, 2016. http://nautil.us. Accessed May 29, 2017.

114. Bonanno GA, Westphal M, Mancini AD. Resilience to loss and potential trauma. *Annual Review of Clinical Psychology*. 2011;7:511–535.

115. Epstein RM, Krasner MS. Physician resilience: What it means, why it matters, and how to promote it. *Academic Medicine: Journal of the Association of American Medical Colleges*. 2013;88(3):301–303.

116. Zwack J, Schweitzer J. If every fifth physician is affected by burnout, what about the other four? Resilience strategies of experienced physicians. *Academic Medicine: Journal of the Association of American Medical Colleges*. 2013;88(3):382–389.

117. Chang J. *Wild Swans: Three Daughters of China*. London, UK: Simon and Schuster; 1991.

118. National Domestic Violence Hotline: 1-800-799-SAFE.

119. Herman J. *Trauma and Recovery: The Aftermath of Violence, from Domestic Abuse to Political Terror*. New York, NY: Basic Books; 1997.

120. Pennebaker J. *Opening Up: The Healing Power of Expressing Emotions*. Rev. ed. New York, NY: Guilford; 1997.

121. Wald HS, Borkan JM, Taylor JS, et al. Fostering and evaluating reflective capacity in medical education: Developing the REFLECT rubric for assessing reflective writing. *Academic Medicine: Journal of the Association of American Medical Colleges*. 2012;87(1):41–50.

122. Charon R, Hermann N. Commentary: A sense of story, or why teach reflective writing? *Academic Medicine: Journal of the Association of American Medical Colleges*. 2012;87(1):5–7.

123. Boyd EM. A reflective learning: Key to learning from experience. *Journal of Humanistic Psychology*. 1983;23:99–117.

124. Miller RE. *Writing at the End of the World*. Pittsburgh, PA: University of Pittsburgh Press; 2005.

125. Driessen E, van Tartwijk J, Dornan T. The self critical doctor: Helping students become more reflective. *British Medical Journal (Clinical Research Edition).* 2008;336(7648):827–830.

126. Mann K, Gordon J, MacLeod A. Reflection and reflective practice in health professions education: A systematic review. *Advances in Health Sciences Education: Theory and Practice.* 2009;14(4):595–621.

127. Talbot J, Rabey S. *The Lessons of St. Francis: How to Bring Simplicity and Spirituality into Your Life.* New York, NY: Penguin; 1998.

128. Kabat-Zinn J. *Mindfulness Mediation for Everyday Life.* London, UK: Biatkus Books; 2001.

129. National Intimate Partner and Sexual Violence Survey. Centers for Disease Control and Prevention. 2017; www.cdc.gov. Accessed November 29, 2017.

130. Clark LT, Ferdinand KC, Flack JM, et al. Coronary heart disease in African Americans. *Heart Disease.* 2001;3(2):97–108.

131. Flack JM, Ferdinand KC, Nasser SA. Epidemiology of hypertension and cardiovascular disease in African Americans. *Journal of Clinical Hypertension.* 2003;5(1 Suppl 1):5–11.

132. Tarver-Carr ME, Powe NR, Eberhardt MS, et al. Excess risk of chronic kidney disease among African-American versus white subjects in the United States: A population-based study of potential explanatory factors. *Journal of the American Society of Nephrology.* 2002;13(9):2363–2370.

133. Douglas JG, Bakris GL, Epstein M, et al. Management of high blood pressure in African Americans: Consensus statement of the Hypertension in African Americans Working Group of the International Society on Hypertension in Blacks. *Archives of Internal Medicine.* 2003;163(5):525–541.

134. Flegal KM, Kit BK, Orpana H, et al. Association of all-cause mortality with overweight and obesity using standard body mass index categories: A systematic review and meta-analysis. *JAMA.* 2013;309(1):71–82.

135. Twig G, Yaniv G, Levine H, et al. Body-mass index in 2.3 million adolescents and cardiovascular death in adulthood. *New England Journal of Medicine.* 2016;374(25):2430–2440.

136. Davis N. Genetic study shows men's height and women's weight drive earning power. *Guardian.* March 8, 2016.

137. Moyer VA. Screening for and management of obesity in adults: U.S. Preventive Services Task Force recommendation statement. *Annals of Internal Medicine.* 2012;157(5):373–378.

138. Sturm R, Hattori A. Morbid obesity rates continue to rise rapidly in the United States. *International Journal of Obesity.* 2013;37(6):889–891.

139. Lanier JB, Bury DC, Richardson SW. Diet and physical activity

for cardiovascular disease prevention. *American Family Physician.* 2016;93(11):919–924.

140. Scherger JE. *Lean and Fit: A Doctor's Journey to Healthy Nutrition and Greater Wellness.* N.p.: CreateSpace Independent; 2016.

141. Rose SA, Poynter PS, Anderson JW, et al. Physician weight loss advice and patient weight loss behavior change: A literature review and meta-analysis of survey data. *International Journal of Obesity.* 2013;37(1):118–128.

142. Lloyd-Jones DM, Hong Y, Labarthe D, et al. Defining and setting national goals for cardiovascular health promotion and disease reduction: The American Heart Association's strategic Impact Goal through 2020 and beyond. *Circulation.* 2010;121(4):586–613.

143. Mosca L, Benjamin EJ, Berra K, et al. Effectiveness-based guidelines for the prevention of cardiovascular disease in women, 2011 update: A guideline from the American Heart Association. *Circulation.* 2011;123(11):1243–1262.

144. Salehi-Abargouei A, Maghsoudi Z, Shirani F, et al. Effects of dietary approaches to stop hypertension (DASH)-style diet on fatal or nonfatal cardiovascular diseases incidence: A systematic review and meta-analysis on observational prospective studies. *Nutrition.* 2013;29(4):611–618.

145. Estruch R, Ros E, Salas-Salvado J, et al. Primary prevention of cardiovascular disease with a Mediterranean diet. *New England Journal of Medicine.* 2013;368(14):1279–1290.

146. Hoevenaar-Blom MP, Nooyens AC, Kromhout D, et al. Mediterranean style diet and 12-year incidence of cardiovascular diseases: The EPIC-NL cohort study. *PLOS One.* 2012;7(9):e45458.

147. *Proceedings from the American Society of Clinical Oncology 2015 Annual Meeting.* Paper presented at the American Society of Clinical Oncology 2015 Annual Meeting; Chicago, IL.

148. Schroeder R, Harrison TD, MCGraw SL. Treatment of adult obesity with bariatric surgery. *American Family Physician.* 2016;93(1):31–37.

149. Ajani UA, Lotufo PA, Gaziano JM, et al. Body mass index and mortality among US male physicians. *Annals of Epidemiology.* 2004;14(10):731–739.

150. Hash RB, Munna RK, Vogel RL, et al. Does physician weight affect perception of health advice? *Preventive Medicine.* 2003;36(1):41–44.

151. Reilly JM. Are obese physicians effective at providing healthy lifestyle counseling? *American Family Physician.* 2007;75(5):738, 741.

152. Brock CD, Stock RD. A survey of Balint group activities in U.S. family practice residency programs. *Family Medicine.* 1990;22(1):33–37.

153. Aviv R. Prescription for disaster: The heartland's pain-pills problem. *New Yorker.* May 5, 2014.

154. Dart RC, Surratt HL, Cicero TJ, et al. Trends in opioid analgesic abuse and mortality in the United States. *New England Journal of Medicine.* 2015;372(3):241–248.

155. Rudd RA, Aleshire N, Zibbell JE, et al. Increases in drug and opioid overdose deaths—United States, 2000-2014. *MMWR Morbidity and Mortality Weekly Report.* 2016;64(50–51):1378–1382.

156. Assessment of pain. American Pain Society. 1996; http://americanpainsociety .org. Accessed December 1, 2017.

157. Weiner RS. *Pain Management: A Practical Guide for Clinicians.* Danvers, MA: CRC; 2001.

158. Cohen S, Doyle WJ, Skoner DP, et al. Social ties and susceptibility to the common cold. *JAMA.* 1997;277(24):1940–1944.

159. Maness DL, Khan M. Nonpharmacologic management of chronic insomnia. *American Family Physician.* 2015;92(12):1058–1064.

160. *International Classification of Sleep Disorders.* 3rd ed. Darien, IL: American Academy of Sleep Medicine; 2014.

161. Cabot JE. *A Memoir of Ralph Waldo Emerson.* Boston, MA: Houghton; 1888.

162. Stress in America 2017: Technology and social media. American Psychological Association. 2017; stressinamerica.org. Accessed July 15, 2017.

163. Moeller SD, Powers E, Roberts J. "The World Unplugged" and "24 Hours without Media": Media literacy to develop self-awareness regarding media. *Scientific Journal of Media Education.* 2012;39:45–52.

164. Sullivan EM, Annest JL, Simon TR, et al. Suicide trends among persons aged 10-24 years: United States, 1994–2012. *MMWR Morbidity and Mortality Weekly Report.* 2015;64(8):201–205.

165. Digital news report. Reuters Institute for the Study of Journalism. University of Oxford. 2016; www.digitalnewsreport.org/. Accessed May 17, 2017.

166. Meeker M. Internet trends 2016: Code conference. Kleiner Perkins. 2016; www.kpcb.com. Accessed May 17, 2017.

167. Marcus M, Yasamy MT, van Ommeren M, et al. *Depression: A Global Public Health Concern.* Washington, DC: WHO Department of Mental Health and Substance Abuse; 2012.

168. Ferrari AJ, Charlson FJ, Norman RE, et al. Burden of depressive disorders by country, sex, age, and year: Findings from the global burden of disease study 2010. *PLOS Medicine.* 2013;10(11):e1001547.

169. Shenk JW. *Lincoln's Melancholy: How Depression Challenged a President and Fueled His Greatness.* New York, NY: Houghton Mifflin Harcourt; 2005.

170. Siu AL, Bibbins-Domingo K, Grossman DC, et al. Screening for depression in

adults: US Preventive Services Task Force recommendation statement. *JAMA.* 2016;315(4):380–387.

171. Maurer DM. Screening for depression. *American Family Physician.* 2012;85(2):139–144.

172. Kroenke K, Spitzer RL, Williams JB. The PHQ-9: Validity of a brief depression severity measure. *Journal of General Internal Medicine.* 2001;16(9):606–613.

173. American Psychiatric Association. *Diagnostic and Statistical Manual of Mental Disorder.* 5th ed. Arlington, VA: American Psychiatric Association Press; 2013.

174. Sullivan GM. The burnout conundrum: Nature versus nurture? *Journal of Graduate Medical Education.* 2016;8(5):650–652.

175. Williams JW, Jr., Gerrity M, Holsinger T, et al. Systematic review of multifaceted interventions to improve depression care. *General Hospital Psychiatry.* 2007;29(2):91–116.

176. Oxman TE, Dietrich AJ, Schulberg HC. The depression care manager and mental health specialist as collaborators within primary care. *American Journal of Geriatric Psychiatry.* 2003;11(5):507–516.

177. Oxman TE, Dietrich AJ, Schulberg HC. Evidence-based models of integrated management of depression in primary care. *Psychiatric Clinics of North America.* 2005;28(4):1061–1077.

178. Ulrich RS. Visual landscapes and psychological well-being. *Landscape Research.* 1979;4(1):17–23.

179. Ulrich RS. Effects of interior design on wellness: Theory and recent scientific research. *Journal of Health Care Interior Design.* 1991;3(1):97–109.

180. Selhub EM, Logan AC. *Your Brain on Nature.* Mississauga, Ontario: Wiley and Sons Canada; 2012.

181. Louv R. *The Nature Principle: Reconnecting with Life in a Virtual Age.* Chapel Hill, NC: Algonquin Books; 2012.

182. Wood H. The John Muir exhibit. Sierra Club. 2017; https://vault.sierraclub .org/john_muir_exhibit. Accessed December 7, 2017.

183. Asch DA, Parker RM. The Libby Zion case: One step forward or two steps backward? *New England Journal of Medicine.* 1988;318(12):771–775.

184. Asch DA, Bilimoria KY, Desai SV. Resident duty hours and medical education policy: Raising the evidence bar. *New England Journal of Medicine.* 2017;376(18):1704–1706.

185. Rigotti NA. Clinical practice: Treatment of tobacco use and dependence. *New England Journal of Medicine.* 2002;346(7):506–512.

186. Pink DH. *Drive: The Surprising Truth about What Motivates Us.* New York, NY: Riverhead Books; 2011.

187. Miller WR, Rollnick S. *Motivational Interviewing: Preparing People for Change.* 3rd ed. New York, NY: Guilford; 2013.

188. Prochaska JO, DiClemente CC. Stages of change in the modification of problem behaviors. *Progress in Behavior Modification.* 1992;28:183–218.

189. Mayer JD, Brackett MA, Salovey P. *Emotional Intelligence: Key Readings on the Mayer and Salovey Model.* Port Chester, NY: Dude; 2004.

190. Goleman D. *Emotional Intelligence: Why It Can Matter More Than IQ.* New York, NY: Bantam Books; 2005.

191. Goleman D, Boyatzis R, McKee A. *Primal Leadership: Unleashing the Power of Emotional Intelligence.* Boston, MA: Harvard Business School; 2013.

192. Kalanithi P. *When Breath Becomes Air.* New York, NY: Random House; 2016.

193. Roosevelt E. *On My Own: The Years since the White House.* New York, NY: Harper and Brothers; 1958.

194. Nattiv A, Loucks AB, Manore MM, et al. American College of Sports Medicine position stand: The female athlete triad. *Medicine and Science in Sports and Exercise.* 2007;39(10):1867–1882.

195. Morgan JF, Reid F, Lacey JH. The SCOFF questionnaire: Assessment of a new screening tool for eating disorders. *British Medical Journal (Clinical research Edition).* 1999;319(7223):1467–1468.

196. Jager AJ, Tutty MA, Kao AC. Association between physician burnout and identification with medicine as a calling. *Mayo Clinic Proceedings.* 2017;92(3):415–422.

197. Careers in medicine. Association of American Medical Colleges. 2015; www.aamc.org/cim/. Accessed May 29, 2017.

198. Krassner P, Adler H, Claus R, et al. An impolite interview with Paul Krassner. *Realist.* 1963;n41(June):24.

199. O'Keefe JH, Bhatti SK, Bajwa A, et al. Alcohol and cardiovascular health: The dose makes the poison . . . or the remedy. *Mayo Clinic Proceedings.* 2014;89(3):382–393.

200. Friedmann PD. Alcohol use in adults. *New England Journal of Medicine.* 2013;368(17):1655–1656.

201. Foroud T, Edenberg HJ, Crabbe JC, et al. Genetic research: Who is at risk for alcoholism. *Alcohol Research and Health.* 2010;33(1–2):64–75.

202. Winslow BT, Onysko M, Hebert M. Medications for alcohol use disorder. *American Family Physician.* 2016;93(6):457–465.

203. Final recommendation statement: Alcohol misuse: Screening and behavioral counseling interventions in primary care. U.S. Preventive Services Task Force. 2013; www.uspreventiveservicestaskforce.org. Accessed December 7, 2017.

204. Lowe E. *Routledge Philosophy Guidebook to Locke on Human Understanding.* London, UK: Routledge; 1995.

205. Rozin P, Royzman EB. Negativity bias, negativity dominance, and contagion. *Personality and Social Psychology Review.* 2001;5(4):296–320.

206. Gottman J, Silver N. *The Seven Principles for Making Marriage Work: A Practical Guide from the Country's Foremost Relationship Expert.* New York, NY: Harmony Books; 2015.

207. Beck AT, Haigh EA. Advances in cognitive theory and therapy: The generic cognitive model. *Annual Review of Clinical Psychology.* 2014;10:1–24.

208. Burns D. *The Feeling Good Handbook.* New York, NY: Penguin; 1999.

209. Grohol JM. 15 Common cognitive distortions. PsychCentral. 2017; http://psychcentral.com. Accessed May 18, 2017.

210. Merton RK. The Thomas Theorem and the Matthew Effect. *Social Forces.* 1995;74(2):379–422.

211. Bowers E. *The Everything Guide to Cognitive Behavioral Therapy.* Avon, MA: Adams Media; 2013.

212. Ellis A. *How to Live with and without Anger: Rational Emotive Therapy, a Revolutionary Technique That Can Improve Your Life.* New York, NY: Reader's Digest Press; 1977.

213. Beck AT. *Cognitive Therapy and the Emotional Disorders.* New York, NY: Penguin; 1979.

214. Coffey SF, Banducci AN, Vinci C. Common questions about cognitive behavior therapy for psychiatric disorders. *American Family Physician.* 2015;92(9):807–812.

215. The Beck learning path. Beck Institute for Cognitive Behavior Therapy. 2016; https://beckinstitute.org/. Accessed May 29, 2017.

216. Souba C. Leading again for the first time. *Journal of Surgical Research.* 2009;157(2):139–153.

217. Souba WW. The science of leading yourself: A missing piece in the health care transformation puzzle. *Open Journal of Leadership.* 2013;2(3):45–55.

218. Centers for Disease Control and Prevention. *CDC Fact Sheet: Incidence, Prevalence, and Cost of Sexually Transmitted Infections in the United States.* 2013. Washington, DC: Centers for Disease Control and Prevention.

219. Lee KC, Ngo-Metzger Q, Wolff T, et al. Sexually transmitted infections: Recommendations from the U.S. Preventive Services Task Force. *American Family Physician.* 2016;94(11):907–915.

220. Van Vranken M. Prevention and treatment of sexually transmitted diseases: An update. *American Family Physician.* 2007;76(12):1827–1832.

221. Hauk L. CDC releases 2015 guidelines on the treatment of sexually transmitted disease. *American Family Physician.* 2016;93(2):144–154.

222. National Health Council. Insurance coverage. Resolve: The National Infertility Association. 2016; www.nationalhealthcouncil.org. Accessed December 7, 2017.

223. Norville D. *Thank You Power: Making the Science of Gratitude Work for You.* Nashville, TN: Nelson; 2007.

224. Fredrickson B. *Positivity: Groundbreaking Research to Release Your Inner Optimist and Thrive.* New York, NY: Crown; 2011.

225. Norris FH, Sloane LB. Epidemiology of trauma and PTSD. In: Friedman MJ, Keane TM, Resick PA, eds. *Handbook of PTSD: Science and Practice.* New York, NY: Guilford; 2007.

226. Winfrey O. *What I Know for Sure.* New York, NY: Harpo; 2014.

227. Fredrickson B. Positive emotions. UNC–Chapel Hill. 2009; www.youtube.com. Accessed December 7, 2017.

# INDEX

Miller, William R., 143
Mindful Attention Awareness Scale
    (MAAS), 16, 17, 25
mindfulness, 15–26; barriers to, 21–22;
    benefits of, 16–17; defined, 15; for
    health-care providers, 17, 22; job
    performance and, 17, 22; learning,
    18–21, 23–24; measurement of, 15–16;
    practice of, 22–26
The Miracle of Mindfulness: An
    Introduction to the Practice of
    Mindfulness (Nhất Hạnh), 20
mission statements, 41, 43
motivational interviewing (MI), 143–44
Motivational Interviewing: Preparing
    People for Change (Miller & Rollnick),
    143
MTF (male to female) transitions, 37
Muir, John, 124
multiple sclerosis (MS), 45
multitasking, 18, 21, 22, 24, 110–12
myocardial infarction. See heart attack

naloxone, 89, 91
narrative writing, 60–63, 65–70
National Domestic Violence Hotline, 58
National Infertility Association, 186
National Institute on Alcohol Abuse
    and Alcoholism, 170
National Intimate Partner and Sexual
    Violence Survey, 67
natural environment, health benefits
    of, 124–25, 133
negativity bias, 96, 172–74
neglect, 4, 83, 127, 146, 160
Neilson, Susie, 47
Nelle (case study), 44–45, 48–53
Nhất Hạnh, Thich, 19, 20
Norville, Deborah, 187–88

nurses. See health-care providers
nurture model of behavior, 171–72
nutrition. See diet and nutrition

obesity, 3, 74–77, 79–81, 104. See also
    weight management
occupational health, defined, 4
Opening Up: The Healing Power of
    Expressing Emotions (Pennebaker), 60
opioids, 90–91, 94, 95
optimism, measurement of, 53
Osler, William, 149
outcomes, factors contributing to,
    174–76, 180–81
overgeneralization, 126, 173, 174
overweight. See obesity
oxycodone, 89–92

pain management, 90–95, 97, 100, 176
Paleolithic diet, 77
patient-doctor relationships, 17, 81–82,
    92–98, 144
Patient Health Questionnaire (PHQ-9),
    120, 121, 123, 126, 128
Peck, M. Scott, 115
pelvic inflammatory disease (PID), 184,
    185
Pennebaker, Jamie, 60
Perez, Johnny, 47
personal balance, 24, 109, 123, 125, 128,
    131
personal health and wellness:
    celebrating progress toward,
    192; challenges and threats to,
    1; in culture of medicine, 8, 130;
    improvement of, 23, 82, 147–50, 192;
    modeling, 84, 125, 129; prioritization
    of, 71; promotion of, 9, 41; self-
    reflection and, 63; sustaining, 151

personal health–improvement tool
(PHIT), 148–50, 192
personalization, 126, 173
personal narratives, 60–63, 65–70
PHIT (personal health–improvement
tool), 148–50, 192
PHQ-9 (Patient Health Questionnaire),
120, 121, 123, 126, 128
physical exercise, 53, 54, 77–79, 83, 121
physical health: alcohol use and,
171; building, 49; complications
involving, 53; defined, 3; education
level and, 7; of health-care providers,
82; social isolation and, 95; stress
and, 121; technology and, 110;
terminal illnesses and, 25
"Physician Resilience: What It Means,
Why It Matters, and How to
Promote It" (Epstein & Krasner), 48
physicians. See health-care providers;
patient-doctor relationships
PID (pelvic inflammatory disease), 184,
185
Pink, Daniel, 143, 157
pneumonia, 50, 52, 138, 140, 185
The Pocket Thich Nhất Hạnh (McLeod),
19, 152
polarized thinking, 172
post-traumatic growth (PTG), 47
post-traumatic stress disorder (PTSD),
47, 104
potentially traumatic events (PTEs), 47
The Power of Mindful Learning (Langer),
17
Primal Leadership: Unleashing the Power
of Emotional Intelligence (Goleman
et al.), 145
Prochaska, James, 143
progress principle, 189

Proust, Marcel, 180
PTEs (potentially traumatic events), 47
PTG (post-traumatic growth), 47
PTSD (post-traumatic stress disorder),
47, 104

rape, 184
reflection, defined, 64–65. See also self-
reflection
reframing thoughts, 176–82
Reid, T. R., 24
religion and spirituality, 3, 15–16, 54, 56
Religious Landscape Study, 3
resilience, 45–54; in adverse situations,
172; assessment of, 48–49, 53–54;
building, 46, 48, 53, 158–59, 177;
definitions of, 45–47; examples of,
48–53; factors contributing to, 47;
promotion of, 3
Resilience: The Science of Mastering Life's
Greatest Challenges (Southwick and
Charney), 48, 158, 159
role models, 7, 23, 54, 128, 160–62, 164
Rollnick, Stephen, 143
Roosevelt, Eleanor, 13, 147
root-cause analysis, 121–22
Roux-en-y gastric bypass procedure,
79–80

Salovey, Peter, 145
Sam (case study), 183–84, 186–87, 191
Sarah (medical student), 55, 57–61, 63,
67–69, 88–89, 92–94, 97
Schweitzer, Albert, vii
Scott, George C., 44
SCOTT five-question tool, 156
self-awareness: components of, 11, 71;
defined, 11; in emotional intelligence
training, 146; health-care providers

and, 58–59; mission and vision statements for, 43; personal narratives as tools for, 63; promotion of, 23; SWOT assessment for, 41–43. *See also* mindfulness

self-care: advancement of, 9, 11; assessment of, 84–86; benefits of, 79, 83–84; challenges of, 81; defined, 71; for health-care providers, 82–83; prioritization of, 20, 191; stigmatization of, 7, 117, 128, 154; strategies for modeling, 130, 131

self-demoralization, 64

self-esteem, 5, 64, 76, 80, 168

self-improvement: assessment of areas for, 131; components of, 71; defined, 135; programs for, 111

self-neglect, 83, 160

self-reflection, 63, 65–67, 69–70

self-SWOT analysis, 41–43, 49, 53, 99

Selhub, Eva, 124

seniors. *See* elderly patients

sexual assault, 184

sexually transmitted infections (STIs), 184–85

Shenk, Joshua Wolf, 119

*She's Not There: A Life in Two Genders* (Boylan), 33

Shirley (case study), 100–109, 112–13

Single Question Screening, 171

Sinsky, Christine, 8

sleep diaries, 104–6

sleep patterns, 100, 102–7, 109, 111–13

SMART goals, 148, 150

smartphones, 110, 111

smoking, 2–3, 59, 82, 87, 139–46, 148–49

social health: alcohol use and, 171; defined, 3–4; technology and, 110; terminal illnesses and, 25

social isolation: assessment of, 96, 98; burnout and, 6, 156; in cycle of power and control, 64; health consequences of, 4, 95–96; interventions for reduction of, 34, 67; suicide and, 33; technology and, 110

social media, 50, 105, 110–11, 146

Social Network Index, 96, 98

social supports, 49, 54, 79, 148

Socrates, 11

Socratic method of inquiry, 29, 41

South Africa: author's work in, 191; resident training with physician from, 81

Southwick, Steven M., 48, 53, 158

spiritual health, defined, 3. *See also* religion and spirituality

stigmatization: of mental-health disorders, 7, 102, 121; obesity and, 76; of self-care, 7, 117, 128, 154; of sexually transmitted infections, 184; suicide and, 33

STIs (sexually transmitted infections), 184–85

stress: biotherapy and, 124; health consequences of, 5, 45, 121; mindfulness practice and, 16–17; pain in relation to, 95; protective factors against, 3; sleep deprivation and, 104; social isolation and, 4, 95–96; technology use and, 110. *See also* chronic stress

stroke, 61, 74, 170, 171

substance abuse, 2, 4–6, 17, 104. *See also* alcohol use; drug use

suicide and suicidal ideation: alcohol use and, 171; burnout and, 6; cyberbullying and, 110; family

member reactions to, 44, 168;
health-care providers and, 66, 154;
intervention programs for, 34;
prevention of, 119–20; risk factors
for, 119, 156; social isolation and,
33; stigmatization and, 33; stress
and, 5

Suzuki, Shunryu, 20–21, 23

SWOT assessment, 41–43, 49, 53, 99, 133

tabula rasa, 171

technology, impact on health, 109–11

*Thank You Power: Making the Science
of Gratitude Work for You* (Norville),
187–88

Thomas Theorem, 174–75

Thoreau, Henry David, 38, 100

throat cancer, 149

time logs, 106–9, 113–15

tobacco use. *See* smoking

transgender patients: counseling for,
40–41; defined, 33; family responses
to, 34–36; gender reassignment
surgery for, 36–37; health concerns
for, 33–34; medical provider
knowledge of, 28–29, 34, 41. *See also*
Carmen (case study)

*Trauma and Recovery* (Herman), 59–60

traumatic experiences, 3, 46, 47, 188

trusting relationships, 64, 91, 93–98

Ulrich, Roger S., 124

United States: alcohol use in, 170;
burnout rates in, 6, 118; depression
rates in, 119; educational disparities
in, 4; health-care spending in, 1; life
expectancy in, 1, 2; mental-health
disorders in, 5; obesity in, 76–77;
opioid epidemic in, 90–91; religion

and spirituality in, 3; sexually
transmitted infections in,
184–85; smartphone usage in,
110

U.S. Preventive Services Task Force,
3, 76, 119–20, 171, 185

Vanderbilt University Wellness Wheel, 3

violence. *See* abuse

Virgil, 165

vision statements, 41, 43

Voltaire, 29

Wasson, John, 86

weight management, 75–77, 80, 83, 86.
*See also* obesity

wellness: in decision-making model,
163–64; defined, 3; evidence-based
initiatives for, 8; modeling, 123, 125,
130, 131, 192; promotion of,
9, 41; threats to, 121, 122, 132.
*See also* personal health and
wellness

Werner, Emmy, 47

*What I Know for Sure* (Winfrey), 188

*When Breath Becomes Air* (Kalanithi), 145

*Wherever You Go, There You Are:
Mindfulness Meditation in Everyday
Life* (Kabat-Zinn), 19–21, 160

WHO (World Health Organization), 2,
3, 19, 119

Winfrey, Oprah, 188

work environment, 4, 122, 125–29

work-life balance, 4, 118, 163

World Health Organization (WHO), 2,
3, 19, 119

World Unplugged Project, 110

*Writing at the End of the World* (Miller),
65

Yerkes, Robert M., 5
yoga, 18, 19, 23, 98
*Your Brain on Nature* (Selhub & Logan), 124
YouTube, 111

*Zen Mind, Beginner's Mind: Informal Talks on Zen Meditation and Practice* (Suzuki), 20–21
Zion, Libby, 128

# ABOUT THE AUTHOR

Dr. Catherine Florio Pipas is a professor of community and family medicine at Dartmouth's Geisel School of Medicine. Over the past twenty-five years she has maintained a family medicine clinical practice. During that time her leadership roles have included assistant dean, vice chair, chief clinical officer, director of the Office of Community-Based Education and Research, and founding director of Dartmouth's Regional Primary Care Center. She has been recognized for excellence in education, research, and clinical care with awards that include 2017 and 2018 NH Top Doctor, Dartmouth Master Educator, Clinical Teacher of the Year, Humanism in Medicine, and AOA Honor Society.

She received her medical degree at Jefferson Medical College and completed residency at Medical University of South Carolina. She earned a Faculty Development Fellowship at UNC–Chapel Hill and an MPH at the Dartmouth Institute for Health Policy and Clinical Practice. Dr. Pipas contributes to the development of undergraduates, medical students, nurses, residents, and faculty across the institution and regionally. She teaches Experiential Public Health and The Culture, Science, and Practice of Wellness at Dartmouth College; directs Dartmouth's Leadership Curriculum; and teaches Applied Leadership for the Leadership Preventive Medicine Residency at Dartmouth Hitchcock Medical Center. She codirects a longitudinal medical school course, Patients and Populations: Improving Health and Healthcare, and provides training in wellness and resilience to promote individual and system-wide improvement that bridges interprofessionals, organizations, and global communities.

She collaborates nationally and internationally to advance her vision for healthy individuals contributing to healthy communities. She serves on the board of directors for the Society of Teachers of Family Medicine and on the board of trustees for Kimball Union Academy and the Association of American Medical Colleges Council of Faculty and Academic Societies.

She is a former president of the New Hampshire Academy of Science and a founding faculty member for STFM's Medical Student Educators Development Institute. She has served on the NH Board of Medicine and contributed to the STFM Leading Change course and the AAMC National LEAD certificate program. She teaches, consults, and collaborates with individuals and organizations, including prehealth, health-care, and public-health professionals. Her areas of interest and expertise include personal health and wellness, personal and professional leadership development, team and systems improvement, community engagement, public health, and population health.